TEST SUCCESS

Test-Taking Techniques for Beginning Nursing Students

TEST SUCCESS

Test-Taking Techniques for Beginning Nursing Students

Patricia M. Nugent, R.N., M.S., Ed.M., Ed.D
Associate Professor, Department of Nursing, Nassau Community College, Garden City, New York

Barbara A. Vitale, R.N., M.A.
Instructor, Department of Nursing, Nassau Community College, Garden City, New York

F. A. DAVIS COMPANY • Philadelphia

Last digit indicates print number: 10 9 8 7 6 5 4 3 2 1

publisher, nursing: **Robert G. Martone**
production editor: **Gail Shapiro**
designer: **Donald B. Freggens, Jr. and Steven R. Morrone**
cover design by: **Donald B. Freggens, Jr.**

As new scientific information becomes available through basic and clinical research, recommended treatments and drug therapies undergo changes. The author(s) and publishers have done everything possible to make this book accurate, up to date, and in accord with accepted standards at the time of publication. The authors, editors, and publisher are not responsible for errors or omissions or for consequences from application of the book, and make no warranty, expressed or implied, in regard to the contents of the book. Any practice described in this book should be applied by the reader in accordance with professional standards of care used in regard to the unique circumstances that may apply in each situation. The reader is advised always to check product information (package inserts) for changes and new information regarding dose and contraindications before administering any drug. Caution is especially urged when using new or infrequently ordered drugs.

Library of Congress Cataloging-in-Publication Data

Nugent, Patricia Mary, 1944-
  Test Success : test-taking techniques for beginning nursing
students / Patricia M. Nugent, Barbara A. Vitale.
    p.   cm.
  Includes bibliographical references and index.
  ISBN 0-8036-6598-9 (alk. paper) :
  1. Nursing--Examinations, questions, etc. 2. Practical nursing-
-Examinations, questions, etc. 3. Test-taking skills. I. Vitale,
Barbara Ann, 1944-   II. Title.
  [DLNM: 1. Educational Measurement. 2. Nursing--examination
questions.   WY 18 N967t]
RT55.N77 1992
610.73'076--dc20
DLNM/DLC
for Library of Congress   92-49452
                                                     CIP

Dedicated To

KELLY MARIE and HEATHER ANN NUGENT

And

JOSEPH MICHAEL, JOHN ANDREW, and CHRISTOPHER NEIL VITALE

for all the joy they have
brought into our lives

Preface

The increase in nursing knowledge and medical technology is accelerating at a breathtaking rate. This places greater stress on nursing students to learn what they need to know to provide safe patient-centered nursing care. Faculty and curricula are stretched to the limit to include all the information students must absorb to successfully complete the requirements to graduate as accountable practitioners. Attrition rates of 12 percent to 30 percent, depending upon the type of nursing program, support the fact that academic demands are strenuous. This is compounded by the fact that nursing students arrive with more needs than ever before. An increasing percentage of nursing students are mature individuals who: have been out of secondary education for years and need to relearn how to study and take tests; are single parents who have the responsibility of supporting children and need to maximize their effectiveness when they study; speak English as their second language and demonstrate needs in reading and/or writing English. In addition, not only are Scholastic Aptitude Test (S.A.T.) scores generally on the decline nationally, but the level of thinking on nursing examinations requires a higher cognitive ability. Beginning nursing students for the first time may be faced with multiple choice questions that require more than just the regurgitation of information but rather the comprehension, application, or analysis of information. Needless to say testing situations induce anxiety for these test takers. Nursing students need supportive textbooks to increase their chances of success.

This book is designed for beginning nursing students who are preparing to take multiple choice tests at the end of a unit of instruction or the completion of a fundamentals of nursing course. Because it takes nursing students at least two years of study to build a body of knowledge upon which safe nursing judgments can be made, this book will only present content common to meeting patient's basic physical and psychosociocultural needs. In addition, content associated with the world of the patient and nurse including such topics as ethics, rights, common theories, legal issues, the nursing process, and principles related to the management of nursing care are also included on a fundamental level. This book can also be used by students or graduates of Licensed Practical Nurse programs to prepare for their national examination or advanced standing examinations for entry into registered nurse programs. In addition, nursing school faculty members can utilize this book to design a test-taking workshop for student nurses.

The chapters of the book are designed to maximize success by presenting techniques that can: empower the learner by promoting a positive mental attitude; increase effectiveness of study effort; instruct the learner to be test wise; and teach the test taker to identify the step in the nursing process being tested to better establish what the question is asking. Six hundred practice questions are provided within the narrative content of Chapters 2 through 5, in three simulated tests in Chapter 6, and in content areas in Chapter

7. All the questions in the book have been field tested and the three simulated tests are designed to have an equal level of difficulty established at 76 percent. The rationales for the correct and incorrect answers are included for each question. These rationales should help the learner review some of the basic content in nursing theory and practice and contribute to mastery of the multiple choice question. The content of questions addresses fundamentals of nursing practice, not intermediate or advanced nursing theory. This book is appropriate for the beginning nursing student, not the student who is preparing for the NCLEX-RN examination.

There are some study guides on the shelves that provide learners with practical skills to become more successful learners. However, no book exists that specifically aids beginning nursing students grappling with the multiple choice question testing fundamental nursing theory and practice. This book was written to fill this void.

We want to thank Tom Manning for his efforts early in the development of this manuscript and Bob Martone who guided and supported us through the publication process. Thanks also go to the F. A. Davis staff including Herbert J. Powell, Jr., Production Manager, Gail Shapiro, Production Editor, Marci Nugent, Copy Editor, Donald B. Freggens, Jr. and Steven R. Morrone, Book Designers. Most importantly, we would like to thank our husbands and children Neil, Kelly, and Heather Nugent and Joe, Joseph, John, and Christopher Vitale for their love and support.

Contents

3 The Multiple-Choice Question

6 Fundamentals of Nursing Practice Tests 113

How to Use this Book to Maximize Success

It is amazing what **you** can achieve when **you** are tenacious, organized, and determined to attain a goal. By purchasing this book **you** have demonstrated a beginning commitment to do what **you** have to do to improve **your** success in multiple choice nursing examinations. This book is designed to introduce **you** to various techniques that can contribute to a positive mental attitude and help **you** become test wise. If you are beginning to get the feeling that "you" is an important word, "you" are right! Learning requires you to be an active participant in your own learning. Your ultimate success can be maximized if you progress through this book in a planned and organized fashion and are willing to practice the techniques suggested. Effort is directly correlated with the benefits you will derive from this book. Once you have determined that you are eager and motivated to learn, then you are ready to begin.

Chapter content is organized in a specific order to provide you with techniques that will contribute to: developing a positive mental attitude; studying and learning more effectively; becoming test wise; and identifying the steps in the nursing process being tested by a question. Six hundred multiple choice nursing questions will afford you the opportunity to practice test-taking techniques. The correct answers and the rationales for all the options are presented to reinforce the theories and principles of fundamentals of nursing practice that you have learned in your nursing program. Three simulated tests of equal difficulty are included to: provide you with a baseline score which reflects your general knowledge of nursing fundamentals and test-taking proficiency; afford you the opportunity to simulate a testing situation; demonstrate successful progress; and motivate you to continue practicing the learned techniques. The simulated tests were placed in Chapter 6 to avoid your inadvertently taking these tests prior to understanding their purpose. To use this book to its best advantage, take one of the simulated tests prior to reading Chapters 1 through 5. This is a pretest because the results will provide you with a baseline score for future comparison. Once you complete Chapters 1 through 5 take another simulated test. Now practice the questions in Chapter 7. Be sure to read and study the rationales because this information will review and reinforce the material you are learning in your fundamentals of nursing course in your school of nursing. To maximize learning, it is suggested that you coordinate answering the questions in the specific categories in Chapter 7 after you learn the content in class. After you finish Chapter 7 take the last of the simulated tests as a post-test. If you are employing the techniques presented in Chapters 1 through 5 and you practice the multiple choice questions in Chapter 7, your test scores should improve from test to test.

It is hard work to take responsibility for your own learning. The magnitude of your learning will be in direct proportion to the amount of energy you are willing to expend in the effort to improve your skills. As you function from a position of strength, study more effectively, become test wise, and are able to apply the nursing process to determine what the question is asking, you should become a more successful test-taker. Good luck on your nursing examinations!

1 Empowerment

Develop a Positive Mental Attitude

A positive mental attitude can help you control test anxiety by limiting anxious responses so that you can be a more successful test-taker. A positive mental attitude requires you to function from a position of strength. This does not imply that you have to be powerful, manipulative, or dominant. What it does require is for you to develop techniques that put you in control of your own thoughts and behavior. To be in control of yourself you need to operate from a position of positive self-worth with a feeling of empowerment.

To develop self-worth, you must be willing to look within yourself and recognize that you are valuable. Acting from a position of strength requires you to start saying and believing that you are worthwhile. Self-worth increases when you believe down to your very bones that you are important.

A feeling of empowerment arises when you are able to use all your available resources and learned strategies to achieve your goals. To achieve empowerment you need to develop techniques and skills that not only make you feel in control but actually position you in control. When you are in control, you function from a position of strength.

To achieve a sense of self-worth and a feeling of empowerment that will help you succeed in test taking, you must learn various techniques that must be practiced prior to taking the test. These learned techniques will help you to control stressful situations, reduce anxious responses, and enhance concentration, thereby improving your analytical and problem-solving ability and strengthening your test performance. By learning and practicing the following techniques, you will have a foundation on which to operate from a position of strength.

Establish an Internal Locus of Control

It is important to recognize that the way you talk to yourself influences the way you think about yourself. The content of what you say indicates how you feel about the control

1

of your behavior and your life. "I was lucky to pass that test." "I couldn't help failing because the teacher is hard." "I got test anxiety and I just became paralyzed during the test." Each of these internal dialogues indicates that you see yourself as powerless. When you say these things, you fail to take responsibility.

Start by identifying your pattern of talking to yourself. Do you blame others, attribute failure to external causes, and use the words "I couldn't," "I should," "I need," or "I have to"? If you do, then you are using language that places you in a position of impotence, dependence, defenselessness, and hopelessness. YOU MUST ESTABLISH AN INTERNAL LOCUS OF CONTROL. You do this by replacing impotent language with language that reflects control and strength. You must say, "I can, I want, and I will." When you use these words, you imply that you are committed to a task until you succeed. Place index cards around your environment with "I CAN," "I WILL," and "I WANT" on them to cue you into a positive pattern of talking to yourself.

Challenge Negative Thoughts

Your value as an individual should not be coupled with how well you do on an examination. Your self-worth and your test score are distinctly isolated entities. If you believe that you are good when you do well on a test and are bad when you do poorly, then you must alter this logic. You need to work at recognizing that this is illogical thinking. Illogical thinking or negative thinking is self-destructive. Negative thinking must be changed into positive thoughts to build confidence and self-worth. As confidence and self-worth rise, anxiety can be controlled and minimized.

Positive thinking focuses your attention on your desired outcomes. If you think you can do well on a test, you are more likely to fulfill this prophecy. It is critical that you control negative thoughts by developing a positive mental attitude. When you say to yourself, "This is a hard test. I'll never pass," CHALLENGE THIS STATEMENT. Instead say to yourself, "This is a ridiculous statement; of course I can pass it. All I have to do is study hard to pass this test!" It is crucial that you challenge negative thoughts with optimistic thoughts. Optimistic thoughts are valuable because they can be converted into positive actions and feelings which place you in a position of control.

For this technique to work, a person must first be able to stop one's thoughts. Use the words ARREST NEGATIVE THOUGHTS. This symbolizes that you will stop these thoughts in their tracks. To do this, you must first identify the pattern of negative thinking that you use as a defense to distract yourself. Envision a police car with flashing lights that signifies ARREST NEGATIVE THOUGHTS. You could even place pictures of police cars around your environment to cue you to ARREST NEGATIVE THOUGHTS. Once you identify negative thoughts, handcuff them and lock them away so they will no longer be a threat. Actually envision negative thoughts locked up in a cell with bars and throw away the key.

Once you stop a negative thought, replace it with a POSITIVE THOUGHT. If you have difficulty identifying a positive thought, praise yourself or give yourself a compliment. Tell yourself, "Wow! I am really working hard to pass this test." "Congratulations! I was able to arrest that negative thought and to be in control." To increase your control, make an inventory of the things you can do, the things you want to achieve, and the feelings you want to feel that contribute to a positive mental attitude. Throughout the day take an "attitude inventory." Identify the status of your mental attitude. If it is not consistent with your list of the feelings you want to feel or the positive image you have of yourself, CHALLENGE THIS ATTITUDE. Compose statements that support the feelings that you want to feel and read them over and over. "I can pass this test!" or "I am in control of my attitudes, and my attitudes are positive!" Make sure that you end the day with a positive thought, and even identify an expectation that you want to accomplish the next day. When you forecast positive events, it establishes a positive direction in which you can focus your attention.

Use Controlled Breathing

An excellent way to reduce feelings of anxiety is to utilize the technique of controlled breathing. When you control your breathing, you can break the pattern of shallow short breaths associated with anxious feelings. Deep abdominal or diaphragmatic breathing enhances the relaxation response. When a person exhales, tense muscles tend to relax. Diaphragmatic breathing causes the diaphragm to flatten and the abdomen to enlarge on inspiration. On exhalation the abdominal muscles contract. As you slowly let out this deep breath, muscles will tend to let go and relax. This technique enables you to breathe more deeply than if you just expand your chest on inspiration. Controlled breathing can be helpful to reduce anxious responses that occur at the beginning of a test, when stumped with a tough question, or when you are nearing the end of the test. During these critical times you can use controlled breathing to induce the relaxation response.

While practicing diaphragmatic breathing, place your hands lightly over the front of the lower ribs and upper abdomen so you can monitor the movement you are trying to achieve. As you become accomplished in this technique you will no longer need to position your hands on the body. Practice the following steps:

1. Gently position your hands over the front of the lower ribs and upper abdomen.
2. Exhale gently and fully. Feel your ribs and abdomen sink inward toward the middle of the body.
3. Slowly inhale a deep breath through your nose allowing the abdomen to expand first and then the chest. Do this as you slowly count to 4.
4. Hold your breath at the height of inhalation as you count to 4.
5. Exhale fully by contracting the abdominal muscles and then the chest. Let out all the air slowly and smoothly through the mouth as you count to 8.

Monitor the pace of your breathing. It is important not to do this exercise too forcefully or too rapidly because it can cause you to hyperventilate. Hyperventilation precipitates dizziness and lightheadedness. Monitor your body. Focus on the muscle group as you inhale and exhale. You may feel warm, tingly, and relaxed. Enjoy the feeling as you breathe deeply and evenly. You should practice this technique so that controlled breathing automatically induces the relaxation response after several breaths. Once you are able to induce the relaxation response with controlled breathing, you can effectively draw upon this strategy when you need to be in control.

Desensitize Yourself to the Fear Response

Individuals generally connect a certain feeling with a specific situation. Controlling feelings requires you to recognize how you consider and visualize events. It is not uncommon to connect a feeling of fear with an event. In a testing situation, the examination is the event and the response of fear is the feeling. If that happens to you, then you need to interrupt this fear response. You have the ability to control how you respond to fear. When you are able to sever the event from the feeling, then you will establish control and become empowered. However, establishing control does not automatically happen. You need to desensitize yourself to the event to control the fear response.

Desensitization involves repeatedly exposing yourself to the identified emotionally distressing event in a limited and/or controlled setting until the event no longer precipitates the feeling of fear. Desensitization is dependent upon associating relaxation with the fear response. To achieve this response, you need to practice the following routine:

FIRST, you must practice a relaxation response. Controlled breathing is an excellent relaxation technique and has already been described. Once you are comfortable with the technique of controlled breathing, you can use it in the desensitization routine.

SECOND, you should make a list of five events associated with a testing situation that cause fear, and rank them starting with the one that causes the most anxiety progressing to the one that causes the least anxiety. The following is an example:

1. Taking an important examination on difficult material
2. Taking an important examination on material you know well
3. Taking a small quiz on difficult material
4. Taking a small quiz on material you know well
5. Taking a practice test that does not count

Event number 5 should invoke the least amount of fear.

THIRD, you should practice the following routine:

- Practice controlled breathing and become relaxed.
- Now imagine event number 5. If you feel fearful, then turn off the scene and go back to controlled breathing for about 30 seconds.
- Once you are relaxed, again imagine scene number 5. Try to visualize the event for 30 seconds without becoming uncomfortable.
- Once you have accomplished the previous step, move up the list of events until you are able to imagine event number 1 without feeling uncomfortable.

When you are successful in controlling the fear response in the testing situation, you can attempt to accomplish the same success in simulated tests at home. Once you are successful in controlling the fear response in simulated tests at home, you can take some simulated tests in a classroom setting. Continue practicing desensitization until you have a feeling of control in an actual testing situation.

Another way you can utilize the concept of desensitization is to practice positive dialogue within yourself. For example, imagine the following internal dialogue with yourself:

"How are you feeling about the examination today?"   "A little uncomfortable and fearful."

"Do you want to feel this way?"   "Absolutely not!"

"How do you want to feel?"   "I want to feel calm, in control, and effective."

"What are you going to do to achieve that feeling?"

"I am going to practice relaxation and controlled breathing."

You might be saying to yourself, "I don't see myself doing this. This is silly." The resilient and tenacious individual who is flexible and willing to try new techniques is in a position of control. If your goal is to be empowered, you only have to be open and willing to learn.

Perform Muscle Relaxation

This technique involves learning how to tense and relax each muscle group of your body until all muscle groups are relaxed. This technique requires practice. The basic technique involves assuming a comfortable position and then sequentially contracting and relaxing each muscle group in your body from the head to the toes. When a muscle group is tensed and then released, the muscle smooths out and relaxes. It is not a technique that can be quickly described in a short paragraph. However, the following brief exercise is included as an example:

EXAMPLE

Find a comfortable chair in a quiet place. Close your eyes and use diaphragmatic breathing taking several deep breaths to relax. You are now ready to begin progressive muscle relaxation. Sequentially move from one muscle group in the body to another, contracting and relaxing each in an even manner. Contract and relax each muscle group for 10 seconds. After each muscle group is tensed and then relaxed, take a deep slow breath using diaphragmatic breathing. As you are relaxing, observe how you feel. Experience the sensation. You may want to reinforce the feeling of relaxation by saying, "My muscles are relaxing. I can feel the tension flowing out of my muscles." Remember not to breathe too forcefully to avoid hyperventilation. The following is a sample of muscle groups that should be included in a progressive muscle relaxation routine:

- Bend your head and try to rest your right ear as close as you can to your right shoulder. Count to 10. Assume normal alignment, relax and take a deep breath.
- Bend your head and try to rest your left ear as close as you can to your left shoulder. Count to 10. Assume normal alignment, relax and take a deep breath.
- Flex your head and try to touch your chin to your chest. Count to 10. Assume normal alignment, relax and take a deep breath.
- Hyperextend your head as far back as it can comfortably hyperextend. Count to 10. Assume normal alignment, relax and take a deep breath.
- Make a fist and tense the right forearm. Count to 10. Relax and take a deep breath.
- Make a fist and tense the left forearm. Count to 10. Relax and take a deep breath.
- Tense the right biceps by tightly bending (flexing) the right arm at the elbow. Count to 10. Relax and take a deep breath.

Continue moving from the head to the arms, trunk, and legs by contracting and relaxing each of the muscle groups within these areas of the body. You can understand and master this technique by obtaining an audio or videotape that is designed to direct and instruct you through the entire routine of tensing and relaxing each muscle group. This technique should be practiced every day over a period of time so that the technique becomes natural. Once you have mastered this technique, you can use a shortened version of progressive relaxation along with controlled breathing at critical times during a test.

Utilize Imagery

Images can establish a state of relaxation. When we remember a fearful event, our heart and respiratory rates increase just as they did when the event occurred. Comparably, when we recall a happy, relaxing period, we can regenerate and re-create the atmosphere and feeling that we had during that pleasant event. This is not a difficult technique to master. Just let go and enjoy the experience.

Position yourself in a comfortable chair, close your eyes, and construct an image in your mind of a place that makes you feel calm, happy, and relaxed. It may be at the seashore or in a field of wild flowers. Let your mind picture what is happening. Observe the colors of the landscape. Notice the soothing sounds of the environment. Notice the smells in the air, the shapes of objects, and movement about you. Recall the positive feelings that flow over you when you are in that scene and relax. You can now open your eyes relaxed, refreshed, and calm.

At critical times during a test, you can take a few minutes to use imagery to induce the relaxation response. To successfully reduce stress, you must position yourself in control. When you are in control, your test performance generally improves.

Overprepare for a Test

One of the best ways to reduce test anxiety is to be overprepared. The more prepared you are to take the test, the more confident you will be. The more confident you are, the more able you are to challenge the fear of being unprepared. Study the textbook, read your notes, take practice tests, and prepare with other students in a study group. Even when you think that you know the information, study the same information again to reinforce your learning. For this technique to be successful, you need to plan a significant amount of time for studying. While it is time-consuming, it does build confidence and reduce anxiety. No one has said learning would be easy. Any worthwhile goal deserves the necessary effort to achieve success. Being overprepared is the BEST way to place yourself in a position of strength.

Consider the following scenario: A student was not doing well in school and asked what she could do to improve her performance. The concept of being overprepared was discussed, and she worked out a study schedule to follow prior to the test. After the test, the student said she thought she did well because the test was an easy test. It had to be pointed out that the test was perceived as easy because she had attained the knowledge that enabled her to correctly answer the questions. Her eyes lit up as if someone turned on a light bulb in her head! When you recognize that you have the opportunity to be in control and take responsibility for your own learning, then you become all that you can be.

Engage in Regular Exercise

Regular exercise assists you to expend nervous energy. Walking, aerobics, swimming, bike riding, or running at least three times a week for 20 minutes is an effective way to maintain or improve your physical and mental status. The most important thing to remember about regular exercise is that you want to slowly increase the degree and duration of the exercise. Your exercise program should not be so rigorous that it leaves you exhausted. It should serve to clear your mind, make you mentally alert and better able to cope with the challenge of a test. Regular exercise should become a routine activity in your weekly schedule, not just a response to the tension of an upcoming test. Once you establish a regular exercise program, you should experience physical and psychological benefits.

ESTABLISHING CONTROL BEFORE AND DURING THE TEST

When you challenge negative thoughts, utilize language that reflects control, are overprepared, rely on desensitization, and use controlled breathing and imagery to induce the relaxation response, you will be functioning from a position of empowerment. It is important to maximize opportunities to feel in control in the testing situation. Additional techniques you can use to establish a tranquil and composed atmosphere require you to take control of your testing equipment, activities before and during a test, and your immediate physical space. Techniques to help create this atmosphere are reinforced in Chapter 5, Test-Taking Strategies. However, they are also discussed here because they can be utilized to reduce anxiety and promote empowerment.

Manage Your Daily Routine Before the Test

It is important to maintain your usual daily routine the day before the test. Eat normally but avoid beverages with caffeine. Caffeine can lessen attention span and reduce concentration by overstimulating your metabolism. Go to bed at your regular time and avoid the urge to stay up late. Implementing usual routines can be relaxing and can contribute to a feeling of control.

Manage Your Study Habits Before the Test

Do not stay up late cramming the night before the big test. Squeezing in last-minute studying may increase anxiety and contribute to feelings of powerlessness and helplessness. If you have implemented a study routine in preparation for the test, you should have confidence in what you have learned. Establish control by saying to yourself, "I have studied hard for this test and I am well prepared. I can relax tonight because I know the material for the test tomorrow and I will do well." Avoid giving in to the desire to cram. Instead, utilize the various techniques discussed earlier in this chapter to maintain a positive mental attitude.

Manage Your Travel the Day of the Test

Plan to arrive early the day of the test. It is important to plan for potential events that could delay you such as traffic jams or a flat tire. The more important the test, the more time you should schedule for transit. If you live a substantial distance from the testing site, you might ask another student who lives closer to allow you to sleep over the night before the test. The midterm or final exam for a course may be held in a different location than the regularly scheduled classroom used for the lecture. If you are unfamiliar with the examination room, make a dry run to locate where it is and note how long it takes to get there. Nothing produces more anxiety than rushing to a test or arriving after the start of a test. A feeling of control reduces tension and the fear response. You can be in control if you manage your travel time with time to spare.

Manage the Supplies You Need for the Test

The more variables you have control over, the more calm and relaxed you will feel. Compose a list of the items you want to bring with you to the test. It may include pencils, pens, scrap paper, erasers, a ruler, something to snack on, or even a lucky charm. It is suggested that you collect the items the day before the test. This eliminates a task that you do not have to worry about on the day of the test and contributes to your sense of control.

Manage the Test Environment

When you arrive early, you generally have the choice of where to sit in the room. This contributes to a feeling of control because you are able to sit where you are most comfortable. It helps to sit near the administrator of the test. Directions may be heard more clearly, and the administrator's attention may be gained more easily if you need to ask a question. Measures that help you feel in control contribute to a positive mental attitude.

Maintain a Positive Mental Attitude

Remind yourself of how hard you worked and how well prepared you are to take this test. ESTABLISH CONTROL by arresting negative thoughts and focusing on the positive. Say to yourself, "I am ready for this test! I will do well on this test! I can get an A on this test!" These statements support a positive mental attitude and enhance a feeling of control.

Manage Your Physical and Emotional Responses

At critical times during the test, you may feel nervous, your breathing may become rapid and shallow, or you may draw a blank on a question. Stop and take a minibreak. Use controlled breathing to induce the relaxation response. You may also use a shortened version of progressive relaxation exercises to induce the relaxation response. Daily practice of breathing and relaxation exercises will enable you to quickly induce the relaxation response during times of stress. Once these techniques are implemented, you should again feel empowered.

SUMMARY

The techniques in this chapter are designed to increase your mastery over the stress of the testing situation. When you feel good about yourself, have a strong self-image, and have a feeling of self-worth, you will develop a sense of control. When you are able to draw upon various techniques that empower you to respond to the testing situation with a sense of calm, you will improve your effectiveness. Use these techniques along with the other skills suggested in this book, practice the questions and then take the simulated practice tests. These activities will support your self-worth, provide you with a feeling of control, and increase your effectiveness in the testing situation.

2 Study Techniques

Learning is the activity by which knowledge, attitudes, and/or skills are acquired. Learning is an exceedingly complex activity that is influenced by various factors such as genetic endowment, level of maturation, experiential background, effectiveness of formal instruction, self-image, readiness to learn, level of motivation, and extent of self-study. Although some of these factors are unchangeable, others are within your ability to control.

Learning is an active process that takes place within the learner. Therefore, the role of the learner is to participate in or initiate activities that promote learning. Like test-taking skills, the ability to effectively learn is not an innate skill. Learning is a learned skill. This chapter presents both general and specific study techniques that should increase your ability to learn. The general study techniques to be presented include skills that facilitate learning regardless of the topic being studied. The specific study techniques are presented in relation to levels of thinking processes that are required to answer multiple-choice questions in nursing: knowledge, comprehension, application, and analysis. Utilization of these techniques when studying will help you to comprehend more of what you have studied and retain the information for a longer period of time. This foundation of information should increase your success in answering multiple-choice questions.

GENERAL STUDY TECHNIQUES

Establish a Routine

Set aside a regular time to study. Learning requires consistency, repetition, and practice. Deciding to sit down to study is the most difficult part of studying. We generally tend to procrastinate and think of a variety of things we must do instead of studying. By committing yourself to a regular routine, you eliminate the repetitive need to make the decision to study. If you decide that every night from 7:00 P.M. to 8:30 P.M. you are going to study, you are utilizing your internal locus of control and establishing an internal readiness to learn. You must be motivated in order to learn.

The study schedule must be reasonable and realistic. Shorter, frequent study periods are more effective than long study periods. For most people, 1- to 3-hour study periods with a 10-minute break each hour are most effective. Periods of learning must be balanced with adequate rest periods because energy and endurance decrease over time and limit learning efficiency. Physical and emotional rest make you more alert and receptive to new information.

When planning a schedule, involve significant family members in the decision making. Because a family is an open system, the action of one family member will influence the other family members. If they are involved in the decision making, they will have a vested interest and probably be more supportive of your adherence to the schedule.

Set Short- and Long-Term Goals

A goal is an outcome that a person attempts to attain and may be long-term or short-term. A long-term goal is the eventual desired outcome. A short-term goal is a desired outcome that can be achieved along the path leading to the long-term goal. In other words, a long-term goal is your destination while the short-term goal is the objective that must be attained to help you eventually reach your destination. Each long-term goal may have one or more short-term goals. Goals should be formulated to promote learning that is purposeful, serve as guides for planning action, and establish standards so that learning can be evaluated. Goals must be specific, measurable, realistic, and have a time frame. A specific goal states exactly what is to be accomplished. A measurable goal sets a minimum acceptable level of performance. A realistic goal must be potentially achievable. A goal with a time frame states the time parameters in which the goal will be achieved. A typical long-term goal would be to correctly answer 90 percent of the study questions at the end of Chapter 1 in the fundamentals of nursing textbook within 7 hours. Typical short-term goals might be: to read and highlight important information in Chapter 1 within 2 hours; to list the principles of nursing practice presented in Chapter 1 within 1 hour; and to compare and contrast information in class notes with information in the textbook within 2 hours. Each of these short-term goals can be achieved as a step toward attaining the long-term goal. It is wise to break a big task into small manageable tasks because it is easier to learn small bits of information than large blocks of information. The most effective learning is goal-directed learning because it is planned learning with a purpose. In addition, when goals are attained, they increase self-esteem and escalate motivation.

Simulate a School Environment

The familiar is generally less stressful than the unfamiliar. Therefore, your posture, surroundings, and equipment should mimic the school or testing environment. Study at a desk or table and chair. Avoid the temptation to study in a reclining chair, on the couch, or in bed. If you are too comfortable you may become complacent or even fall asleep. Gather all the necessary equipment for studying such as your textbook, class notes, paper, pens, a highlighter, a dictionary, and so on. Use the same tools you plan to use when you take your examinations. Control other factors that reflect the testing environment such as ensuring adequate light or avoiding eating while you are studying. The study environment should be comfortable enough to promote learning while stringent enough to prevent apathy, indifference, or nonchalance.

Control Internal and External Distractors

Stimuli, both internal and external, must be controlled to eliminate distractions. External stimuli are environmental happenings that interrupt your thinking and should be limited. Select a place to study where you will not be interrupted by family members, phone calls, the doorbell, or family pets. Do not study while watching television or listening to the radio. These stimuli compete for your attention when you need to be focusing on your work. Internal stimuli are your inner thoughts, feelings, or concerns that interfere with your ability to study. Internal stimuli are often more difficult to control than external stimuli because they involve attitudes. Review the techniques in Chapter 1 that promote a positive mental attitude. By limiting or eliminating internal and external distractors, you should improve your ability to concentrate.

Utilize a Variety of Learning Methods

Learning is the process by which you attain new information, acquire new skills, or formulate new attitudes. New information is usually learned through symbols such as words or pictures. We read them, see them, or hear them. Use all your senses to maximize your acquisition and comprehension of new information. The more routes that information can transverse to reach your brain, the greater the chances are that you will learn the information. For example, when reading information about the stages of decubitus ulcers, learning is reinforced by viewing pictures of the various stages of decubitus ulcers.

New skills involve the physical application of information. It is possible for a person to understand all the goals and steps of a procedure and yet not be able to perform the procedure. For information to get from the head to the hands, the learner must do more than read a book, look at pictures, view a video, or watch other people. The learner must become actively involved. Skills are not learned by osmosis; they are learned by "doing." For example, when learning how to perform range of motion to a hand, the learner can read a book and look at pictures, but the learner must actually practice moving a person's hand through range of motion.

Learning new attitudes represents an increasing internalization or commitment to a feeling, belief, or value. This is the most difficult type of learning because attitudes result from lifelong learning and tend to be well entrenched. In addition, the attainment of new attitudes is difficult to evaluate. For example, a student nurse may know and understand the theory concerning why nurses should be nonjudgmental and yet in a clinical situation may be judgmental toward the patient. New attitudes are best developed within an atmosphere of acceptance and by exploring feelings, becoming involved in group discussions, and observing appropriate role models. For example, prior to providing perineal care for the first time, it is beneficial for student nurses to explore feelings about invading a patient's personal space.

How we learn is never identical for two different people, nor is it identical for one person in different situations. Over the years you have developed a learning style with which you feel comfortable and which has proven successful. However, be open to a variety of learning approaches.

Capture Moments of Time

Utilizing spare moments is a method of maximizing your time for constructive study. All humans have periods of time during the day that are less productive than others such as waiting at a red light or standing in line at a store. Also there are times that you engage in repetitive tasks such as vacuuming a rug or raking the leaves. Capture these moments of time and exploit them. Carry flash cards, a vocabulary list, or categories of information that you can contemplate when you have unexpected time. These captured moments should be an adjunct to, rather than replace, your regularly scheduled study periods. There is an old adage that states, *"Time is on your side."* Capture spare moments of time and employ them to your advantage.

Utilize Appropriate Resources

The theories and principles of nursing practice are complex. They draw from a variety of disciplines (psychology, sociology, anatomy and physiology, microbiology, and so on), use new terminology, and require unique applications to clinical practice. When studying, learning does not occur on a straight line aimed forward and upward. You may experience plateaus, remissions, and/or periods of confusion when dealing with complex material. When your forward progress is stymied, identify your needs and immediately seek help. Your teacher, another student, a study group, or a tutor may be beneficial. When studying with another student, ensure that the person is a reliable source of correct information. When studying in groups, three to five students is ideal because a group of more than five people becomes a "party." The group should be heterogeneous; that is, there should be a variety of academic abilities, attitudes, skills, and perspectives among the participants. This variety should enrich the learning experience and provide checks and balances for the sharing of correct information. To utilize appropriate resources, you must be willing to be open to yourself and others. Have the courage to acknowledge to yourself and others that you need assistance and then be receptive to the sharing process. You learn not only from the instructor but from yourself and your classmates.

Balance Sacrifice and Rewards

When you decided to enter nursing school, no one ever promised you a rose garden. Your commitment to becoming a nurse requires sacrifice. Your time and energy are being diverted away from your usual activities related to a job, family members, friends, or pleasurable pastimes. To manage your time and responsibilities efficiently and fairly, you may have to make difficult decisions. Reducing work hours, sharing household chores, hiring a baby sitter, or limiting your social life may be necessary strategies to help you attain your goal of becoming a nurse. Avoid overextending yourself because if you do, you will be setting yourself up for failure. The reality is that the course of study in nursing school is rigorous and it will command most of your time and energy.

Rigorous activity, whether it be physical or mental, requires concentration and endurance. However, too much work hinders productivity. You must establish a balance between energy expenditure and rewards for your efforts. Rewards can be internal or external. Internal rewards are stimulated from within the learner and relate to feelings associated with meaningful achievement. Learning something new, achieving a goal, or increasing self-respect are examples of internal rewards. External rewards arise from outside the learner. A grade of 100 percent, respect and appreciation from others, or a present for achieving a goal are examples of external rewards. Unfortunately, the rewards for studying are usually not immediate but rather in the extended future. Graduating from nursing school, passing the NCLEX-RN examination, earning a paycheck, and enjoying the prestige of being a nurse are future-oriented rewards. Therefore, you should be the one to provide immediate rewards for yourself for studying. During study breaks or at the completion of studying, reward yourself by thinking about how much you have learned, reflecting on the good feelings you have about your accomplishments, relaxing with a significant other, having a cup of coffee, watching a favorite television show, calling a friend on the telephone, or taking a weekend off. Short-term rewards promote a positive mental attitude, reinforce motivation, and provide a respite from studying.

SPECIFIC STUDY TECHNIQUES

Cognitive Levels of Nursing Questions

The nurse utilizes a variety of thinking processes when caring for patients. Therefore, nursing examinations must reflect these thinking processes to effectively evaluate the safe practice of nursing. There are four types of thinking processes that are incorporated into multiple-choice questions concerning the delivery of nursing care: *knowledge, comprehension, application,* and *analysis.* These thinking processes are within the cognitive domain ("understanding information") and are ordered on the concept of complexity of behavior. That is, a knowledge question requires the lowest level of thinking (recalling information) while an analysis question requires the highest level of thinking (comparing and contrasting information).

In this section of the book each cognitive level (knowledge, comprehension, application, and analysis) is discussed, and sample items are presented to illustrate the thinking processes involved in answering the item. In addition, specific study techniques are presented to help you to strengthen your thinking abilities and learn new information.

For your information the correct answers for the sample items in this chapter and the rationales for all the options are at the end of this chapter.

Knowledge Questions

Knowledge questions require you to recall or remember information. To answer a knowledge question, you need to commit facts to memory. Knowledge questions expect you to know terminology, specific facts, trends, sequences, classifications, categories, criteria, structures, principles, generalizations, or theories.

SAMPLE ITEM 2–1

When administering medications, *qid* means:

(1) Once a day
(2) Twice a day
(3) Three times a day
(4) Four times a day

To correctly answer this question, you have to know the meaning of the abbreviation *qid.*

SAMPLE ITEM 2–2

The first step of the procedure for making an unoccupied bed is:

(1) Washing the hands

(2) Pulling the curtain

(3) Collecting clean linen

(4) Placing the bottom sheet

To correctly answer this question, you need to know the sequence of steps in the procedure of making an unoccupied bed or the basic principle that the hands must be washed prior to care.

SAMPLE ITEM 2–3

What is the normal range of a radial pulse in an adult?

(1) 50 to 65

(2) 70 to 85

(3) 90 to 105

(4) 110 to 125

To answer this question correctly, you have to know the normal range of a radial pulse in an adult.

Memorization by Repetition

Knowledge questions require you to remember information that forms the foundation of nursing practice. Initially, information can be learned by memorization. Memorization is committing information to the brain through repetition for recall at a later time. Repeatedly studying information by reciting it out loud, reviewing it in your mind, or writing it down increases your chances of remembering the information because a variety of senses is employed. Memorization can be facilitated by the use of lists of related facts, flash cards, or learning wheels. For example:

- On an index card you can list the steps of a procedure. This can be carried with you to study when you capture moments of time.

- On the front of an index card you can write a word and on the back define the word. Develop an entire deck of cards that relates to the terminology within a unit of study. Again, use the flash cards when you have unexpected time to study.

- To make a learning wheel, cut a piece of cardboard into a circle and draw pie shaped wedges on the front and back. On a front wedge write a unit of measure, such as 30 ml, and on the corresponding back wedge write its conversion to another unit of measure, such as 1 ounce. Then on individual spring clothespins, write each of the units of measure that appear on the backside of the wheel. When you want to study approximate equivalents, mix up the clothespins and attempt to match each one to its corresponding unit of measure. You can turn the wheel over and evaluate your success by determining if the clothespin you attached to the wheel matches the unit of measure on the back of the wheel.

These memorization techniques reinforce learning by the use of repetition, but the information is learned by rote memorization without any in-depth understanding of the information learned. Information learned by repetition uses short-term memory and is generally quickly forgotten unless reinforced through additional study techniques or application in your nursing practice.

Alphabet Cues

The memorization of information can be facilitated if the information is associated with letters of the alphabet. Each letter serves as a cue that stimulates the recall of associated information. The most effective alphabet cues are those you formulate yourself. They meet a self-identified need, and you must review the information before you can design the alphabet cue. You can use any combination of letters as long as they have significance for you and your learning. Examples of alphabet cues include:

- The *ABC*s of cardiopulmonary resuscitation are: *Airways*—clear the airway; *Breathing*—initiate artificial breathing; *Circulation*—initiate cardiac compression.

- Identify patients at high risk for injury through the letters *A, B, C, D, E, F, G: Age*—the young and old; *Blindness*—lack of visual perception; *Consciousness*—decreased level of consciousness; *Deafness*—lack of auditory perception; *Emotional state*—reduced perceptual awareness; *Frequency of accidents*—previous history of accidents; and *Gait*—impaired mobility.

- The three Ps for the cardinal signs of diabetes mellitus are: Polyuria, Polydipsia, and Polyphagia.

Acronyms

An acronym is a word formed from the first letters of a series of statements or facts. The acronym itself dynamically relates to the information it represents. It is useful to learning because each letter of the word jostles the memory to recall significant information. An acronym is an effective technique to retrieve previously learned information. Examples of acronyms include the following:

- The American Cancer Society teaches the early warning signs of cancer through the acronym of *CAUTION:*

    *C*hange in bowel and bladder habits

    A sore that does not heal

    *U*nusual bleeding or discharge

    *T*hickening or a lump

    *I*ndigestion or difficulty in swallowing

    *O*bvious change in a wart or mole

    *N*agging cough or hoarseness

- When assessing a patient for adaptations indicating the presence of infection, remember the acronym *INFECT:*

*I*ncreased pulse and respirations

*N*odes are enlarged

*F*unction is impaired

*E*rythema, edema, exudate

*C*omplaints of discomfort or pain

*T*emperature—local and/or systemic

Acrostics

An *acrostic* is a phrase, motto, or verse in which a letter of each word (usually the first letter) prompts the memory to retrieve important information. A variation of an acrostic is a sentence with content that jogs the memory. Memorizing information can be difficult and boring. This technique is a creative approach to make learning more effective and fun. Examples of acrostics include the following:

- When studying the fat-soluble vitamins, recall this motto, "*All Dieters Eat Kilocalories.*" This should help you remember that *A, D, E,* and *K* are the fat-soluble vitamins.

- When studying apothecary and metric equivalents, remember this verse, "There are *15 grains* of sugar in *1 gram* cracker." This sentence should help you remember that *15 grains* are equivalent to *1 gram*.

Comprehension Questions

Comprehension questions require you to understand information. To answer a comprehension question, not only must you commit facts to memory but it is essential that you can translate, interpret, and determine the implications of the information. You demonstrate understanding when you translate or paraphrase information, interpret or summarize information, or determine the implications, consequences, corollaries, or effects of information. Comprehension represents the lowest level of understanding. Comprehension questions expect you to not only know but understand information being tested without necessarily relating it to other material or seeing its fullest implications.

SAMPLE ITEM 2–4

To evaluate the therapeutic effect of a cathartic, the nurse should assess the patient for:

(1) Increased urinary output

(2) A decrease in anxiety

(3) A bowel movement

(4) Pain relief

To answer this question, you not only have to know that a cathartic is a potent laxative that stimulates the bowel but that the increase in peristalsis will result in a bowel movement.

SAMPLE ITEM 2–5

When clarifying is used as a therapeutic communication tool, the nurse is:

(1) Verifying what is implied by the patient

(2) Summarizing the patient's communication

(3) Restating what the patient has said.

(4) Paraphrasing the patient's message

To answer this question, you not only have to know that clarifying is a therapeutic tool that promotes communication between the patient and nurse but you must explain why or how this technique facilitates communication.

SAMPLE ITEM 2–6

After administering an intramuscular injection, the nurse should massage the needle insertion site to:

(1) Limit infection

(2) Prevent bleeding

(3) Reduce discomfort

(4) Promote absorption

To answer this question, you not only have to know that massage is one step of the procedure for an intramuscular injection but you have to understand the consequence of massaging the needle insertion site once the needle is withdrawn.

Explore "Whys" and "Hows"

The difference between knowledge questions and comprehension questions is: to answer knowledge questions, you must know facts; to answer comprehension questions, you must understand the significance of facts. Facts can be understood and retained longer if they are relevant and meaningful to the learner. When studying information, ask yourself "why" or "how" is this information important. For example, when learning that immobility causes decubitus ulcers, explore *why* they occur. Pressure compresses the capillary beds which interferes with the transport of oxygen and nutrients to tissues resulting in ischemia and necroses. When studying a skill such as bathing, explore *why* soap is used. Soap reduces the surface tension of water and helps remove accumulated oils, perspiration, dead cells, and bacteria. If you interpret information and identify *how* or *why* the information gained is relevant and useful, then the information has value. Valued information increases in significance and is less readily forgotten.

Study in Small Groups

Once you have studied by yourself, it is usually valuable to study the same information with another person or in a small group. The sharing process promotes comprehension of information because you listen to the impressions and opinions of others, learn new information from a peer tutor, and reinforce your own learning by teaching others. In addition, the members of the group reinforce your interpretation of information and correct your misunderstanding of information. The value of group work is in the exchange process. Group members must listen, share, evaluate, help, support, reinforce, discuss, and debate to promote learning. There is truth in the adage *"One hand washes the other."* Not only do you help yourself but you help another person.

Application Questions

Application questions require you to utilize knowledge. To answer an application question, you must take remembered and comprehended abstractions and apply them to concrete situations. The abstractions may be theories, technical principles, rules of procedures, generalizations, or ideas which have to be applied in a presented scenario. Application questions test your ability to use information in a new situation.

SAMPLE ITEM 2–7

An elderly patient's skin looks dry, thin, and fragile. When providing back care, the nurse should:

(1) Apply a moisturizing body lotion
(2) Wash the back with soap and water
(3) Massage using short kneading strokes
(4) Leave excess lubricant on the patient's skin

    To answer this question, you must know that dry, thin, fragile skin is common in the elderly and moisturizing lotion helps the skin to retain water and become more supple. When presented with this patient scenario, you have to apply your knowledge concerning developmental changes in the elderly and the consequences of the use of moisturizing lotion.

---

to page 21

SAMPLE ITEM 2–8

When caring for several patients on bladder-retraining programs, the nurse should recognize that an intervention that is always implemented during a bladder-retraining program is toileting:

(1) Every 2 hours when awake

(2) At 8 AM, 2 PM, 8 PM, and 2 AM

(3) When the patient goes to bed at night

(4) Every 4 hours and through the night

To answer this question, you have to understand the principle that nursing care should be individualized. You also must understand the commonalities within the procedure of bladder retraining. When presented with this concrete situation, you have to apply your knowledge about patient-centered care and the theoretical components of bladder-retraining programs.

SAMPLE ITEM 2–9

To prevent self-injury when lifting a heavy patient higher in bed, the nurse should:

(1) Keep the knees and ankles straight

(2) Straighten the knees and bend at the waist

(3) Place the feet together with the knees bent

(4) Position the feet apart with one placed forward

To answer this question you have to understand the principles of body mechanics. You also need to apply these principles in a particular patient care situation, moving a heavy patient higher in bed.

Relate New Information to Prior Learning

Learning is easier when information to be learned is associated with what you already know. Therefore, relate new information to your foundation of knowledge, experience, attitudes, and feelings. For example, when studying the principles of body mechanics, review which principles are utilized when you carry a heavy package, move from a lying-down to a standing position, or assist an elderly relative to walk up a flight of stairs. When studying the principles of surgical asepsis, recall and review the various situations when you performed sterile technique and identify the principles that were the foundation of your actions. Visualizing abstractions, such as principles and theories, being applied in concrete situations reinforce the ability to utilize them in future circumstances.

Recognize Commonalities

The application of information demonstrates a higher level of understanding than just knowing or comprehending information because it requires the learner to show, solve, modify, change, use, or manipulate information in a real situation or a presented scenario. To facilitate learning to apply information, identify commonalities when studying principles and theories that can be used in a variety of situations. A commonality exists when two different situations require the application of the same or similar principle. For example, when studying the principle of gravity, you must understand that it is the force that draws all mass in the earth's sphere toward the center of the earth. Now attempt to identify situations that employ this principle. As a nurse, you apply this principle when you place a urine collection bag below the level of the bladder, hang an intravenous bag higher than the needle insertion site, raise the head of the bed for a patient with dyspnea, and raise the foot of the bed for a patient with dependent edema. This study technique is particularly effective when working in small groups because it involves brainstorming. Others in the group because of their different perspectives may identify situations that you would not consider. Recognizing commonalities reinforces information and maximizes the application of information in patient care situations.

Analysis Questions

Analysis questions require you to interpret a variety of data and recognize the commonalities, differences, and interrelationships among presented ideas. Analysis questions make the assumptions that you know, understand, and can apply information. Now you must identify, examine, dissect, evaluate, or investigate the organization, systematic arrangement, or structure of the information presented in the question. This type of question tests your analytical ability.

SAMPLE ITEM 2–10

A patient has dependent edema of the ankles and feet and is obese. The nurse should expect the physician to order which of the following diets?

(1) Low in salt and high in fat
(2) Low in salt and low in calories
(3) High in salt and high in protein
(4) High in salt and low in carbohydrates

To answer this question, you have to understand the inherent relationships between salt in the diet and fluid retention, and obesity and caloric intake. You also must understand the impact of carbohydrates, proteins, and fats in a diet for a patient with edema and obesity. When you answer this question, you must understand and examine the information presented, identify the interrelationships among elements, and arrive at a conclusion.

SAMPLE ITEM 2–11

A patient who is undergoing cancer chemotherapy says to the nurse, "This is no way to live." Which of the following responses uses reflective technique?

(1) "Tell me more about what you are thinking."
(2) "You sound discouraged today."
(3) "Life is not worth living?"
(4) "What are you saying?"

To answer this question, you must understand the communication techniques of reflection, clarification, and paraphrasing. You also must analyze statements and identify the use of these techniques in presented conversations. This question requires you to understand, interpret, and differentiate information.

SAMPLE ITEM 2–12

The physician orders 500 mg of an antibiotic to be administered via an intramuscular injection. A 1-gram vial of the medication, which needs to be reconstituted, states: Add 2.7 ml of solution to yield 3 ml. How much solution should the nurse administer?

(1) 0.5 ml
(2) 1.0 ml
(3) 1.5 ml
(4) 2.0 ml

To answer this question, you must understand the relationship of milligrams to grams (1000 mg = 1 gram; therefore, 500 mg = 0.5 gram) and use a formula for ratio and proportion. This question requires you to identify the various components within the problem, select the appropriate formula required to solve the problem, place the correct elements within the formula, and then implement the mathematical calculation to arrive at the answer.

Recognize Differences

Analysis questions require an ability to analyze information which is a higher thought process than knowing, understanding, or applying information. For example, when studying blood pressure, you first memorize the parameters of a normal blood pressure (knowledge). Then you develop an understanding of what factors influence and produce a normal blood pressure (comprehension). Then you identify a particular patient situation that would necessitate obtaining a blood pressure (application). Finally, you must differentiate among a variety of situations and determine which has the highest priority for assessing the blood pressure (analysis). Analysis questions are difficult because they demand a scrutiny of all the data presented in the stem and options. Because these questions often require you to use differentiation to determine the significance of information, the recognition of differences among learned information is an effective study technique.

To study for complex questions, you cannot just memorize and understand facts or recognize the commonalities among facts, you must learn to differentiate. When studying the causes of an elevated blood pressure, identify the different causes and why they would result in an increased blood pressure. For example, a blood pressure can rise for a variety of reasons: infection causes an increased metabolic rate; fluid retention causes hypervolemia; and anxiety causes an autonomic nervous system response that constricts blood vessels. In each situation the blood pressure increased but for a different reason. Recognizing differences is an effective study technique to broaden the interrelationship and significance of learned information.

Practice Test Taking

Taking practice tests is an excellent way to improve the effectivess of your test-taking techniques. Not only can you become more emotionally and physically comfortable in the testing situation but you can become more proficient at selecting the correct option when answering a multiple-choice question. Reviewing rationales for the right and wrong answers serves as an effective study technique. It reinforces learning and it can help you identify areas that require additional study.

As you practice test taking, it is advised that you gradually increase the time interval that you spend when taking a practice test. By increasing your practice time to 2- to 3-hour intervals, you can build stamina enabling you to concentrate more effectively during a shorter test. Marathon runners have long recognized the value of building stamina and the need for practice to achieve a "groove" that enhances performance. Marathon runners also manage their practice so they "peak" the day of the big event. The same principles can be applied to the nursing student preparing for an important test. You are at your peak and can achieve a groove when you feel physically, emotionally, and intellectually ready for the important test.

Practicing test taking should assist you to:

Acquire new knowledge

Comprehend information

Apply theories and principles

Utilize test-taking techniques

Understand concepts

Reinforce previous learning

Apply problem-solving skills

Identify rationales for nursing interventions

Analyze information

Identify commonalities and differences in situations

Effectively manage time during a test

Control your environment

Contribute to a positive mental attitude

Control physical and emotional responses

Feel empowered and in control

ANSWERS AND RATIONALES FOR SAMPLE ITEMS IN CHAPTER 2

An asterisk (*) is in front of the rationale that explains the correct answer.

2–1   (1) The abbreviation for once a day is *qd.*
    (2) The abbreviation for twice a day is *bid.*
    (3) The abbreviation for three times a day is *tid.*
    * (4) The abbreviation for four times a day is *qid.*

2–2 * (1) Washing the hands removes microorganisms that can contaminate the clean linen.
    (2) This is unnecessary when making an unoccupied bed; this is required to provide for privacy when making an occupied bed.
    (3) This is done after the hands are washed to prevent contamination of the linen.
    (4) This is done after the hands are washed and the sheets are collected.

2–3   (1) This is below the normal range for the pulse in an adult.
    * (2) This is within the normal range of 60 to 100 beats per minute for the pulse of an adult.
    (3) Although 90 is within the high end of the normal range for the pulse of an adult, the 110 is above the normal range.
    (4) This is above the normal range for the pulse of an adult.

2–4   (1) Diuretics produce an increase in urinary output.
    (2) Antianxiety agents (anxiolytics) reduce anxiety.
    * (3) Cathartics stimulate bowel evacuation; therefore, the patient should be assessed for a bowel movement.
    (4) Analgesics alter the perception and interpretation of pain.

2–5 * (1) Clarifying is a method of making the client's message more understandable; it is an attempt to obtain more information without interpreting the patient's original statement.
    (2) Summarizing reviews the main points in a discussion; this is useful at the end of an interview or teaching session.
    (3) Restating, also called "paraphrasing," is a technique that repeats the patients's basic message in similar words.
    (4) Same as #3.

2–6   (1) Using sterile equipment and sterile technique limits infection.
    (2) Removing the needle along the line of insertion and pressure at the site prevent bleeding.
    (3) Removing the needle along the line of insertion and depressing the skin with a swab while the needle is withdrawn reduce discomfort.
    * (4) Massage disperses the medication in the tissues and facilitates its absorption.

2–7 * (1) Moisturizing lotion limits dryness and reduces friction of the hands against the skin which prevents skin trauma.
    (2) Soap should be avoided because it can further dry the skin.
    (3) This can cause injury to delicate, thin skin and light, long strokes should be used.
    (4) This can promote skin maceration and also provides a warm, moist environment for the growth of microorganisms, which should be avoided.

2–8 (1) This may not be appropriate for all residents; a bladder-retraining program must be based on individual needs.
(2) Same as #1.
* (3) All patients, regardless of the specifics of their own bladder-retraining program, will be toileted before going to bed at night and after awakening in the morning.
(4) Same as #1.

2–9 (1) This places strain on the muscles of the back and should be avoided.
(2) Same as #1.
(3) Keeping the feet together produces a narrow base of support which can result in a fall.
* (4) Both actions provide a wide base of support which promotes stability; placing one foot in front of the other facilitates bending at the knees which permits the muscles of the legs, rather than the back, to bear the patient's weight.

2–10 (1) Although a low-salt diet would be appropriate to limit edema, a diet high in fat should be avoided by an obese individual because fats are high in calories.
* (2) Salt promotes fluid retention and increased calories add to body weight; therefore, both should be avoided by this patient.
(3) Salt promotes fluid retention and should be avoided by this patient; protein is unrelated to this patient's problem.
(4) Although carbohydrates may be restricted in an obese individual to facilitate weight loss, a high-salt diet would promote fluid retention and should be avoided.

2–11 (1) This response is using the technique of clarification and asks the patient to expand on the message so that it becomes more understandable.
* (2) This response is using reflective technique because it attempts to identify feelings within the patient's message.
(3) This response is using the technique of paraphrasing because it restates the patient's basic message in similar words.
(4) Same as #1.

2–12 (1) This is an incorrect calculation and is less than the ordered dosage of medication.
(2) Same as #1.
* (3) When using ratio and proportion, solve for X by cross-multiplying:

$$\frac{0.5 \text{ g (desired dosage)}}{1.0 \text{ g (supplied dosage)}} \quad \frac{X \text{ ml}}{3 \text{ ml}}$$

$$1.0X = 3 \times 0.5$$

$$X = 1.5 \text{ ml}$$

(4) This is an incorrect calculation and is more than the ordered dosage of medication.

3 The Multiple-Choice Question

       In our society success is generally measured in relation to levels of achievement. Prior to entering formal institutions of learning, your achievement was subjectively appraised by your family and friends. Success was rewarded by smiles, positive statements, and perhaps favors or gifts. Lack of achievement or failure was acknowledged by omission of recognition, verbal corrections, and possibly punishment or scorn. When you entered school your performance was directly measured against acceptable standards. In an effort to eliminate subjectivity, you were exposed to objective testing. These tests included true-false questions, matching columns, and multiple-choice questions. Achievement was reflected by numerical grades or letter grades. These grades indicated your level of achievement and by themselves provided rewards and punishments.

       In nursing education, achievement can be assessed in a variety of ways: a patient's physiological response (did the patient's condition improve), a patient's verbal response (did the patient state improvement), student nurses' clinical performance (did the students do what they were supposed to do), and student nurses' levels of cognitive competency (did the students know what they were supposed to know). The *ultimate* written test in nursing is the *National Council Licensing Examination,* also known as NCLEX-RN. It is the ultimate examination because you must successfully pass this test to be licensed to practice nursing. The NCLEX-RN consists entirely of multiple-choice questions. Because of this fact, multiple-choice questions are frequently used in schools of nursing to evaluate student progress throughout the nursing curriculum. They are also utilized because they are objective, time efficient, and can comprehensively assess curriculum content that has depth and breadth. Therefore, it is important for you to understand the components and dynamics of multiple-choice questions early in your nursing education.

       A multiple-choice question is an objective test item. It is objective because the perceptions or opinions of another person do not influence the grade. In a multiple-choice question, a question is asked, three or more potential answers are presented, and only one of the potential answers is correct. Either the student answers the question correctly or not.

COMPONENTS OF A MULTIPLE-CHOICE QUESTION

The entire multiple-choice question is called an *item.* Each item consists of two parts. The first part is known as the *stem.* The stem is the statement that asks the question. The second part contains the possible responses offered by the item, which are called *options.* One of the options answers the question posed in the stem and is the *correct answer.* The remaining options are the incorrect answers and are called *distractors.* They are referred to as "distractors" because they are designed to distract you from the correct answer.

The correct answers and the rationales for all the options of the sample items are at the end of this chapter. Test yourself and see if you can correctly answer the sample items.

SAMPLE ITEM 3–1

Before performing any patient procedure, the nurse should first plan to:

(1)	Shut the door	DISTRACTOR
(2)	Wash the hands	CORRECT ANSWER
(3)	Close the curtain	DISTRACTOR
(4)	Drape the patient	DISTRACTOR

S T E M — STEM
O P T I O N S — OPTIONS
I T E M

SAMPLE ITEM 3–2

When providing care to a patient with a nasogastric tube, the nurse recognizes that the tube goes into the:

(1)	Stomach	CORRECT ANSWER
(2)	Bronchi	DISTRACTOR
(3)	Trachea	DISTRACTOR
(4)	Duodenum	DISTRACTOR

S T E M — STEM
O P T I O N S — OPTIONS
I T E M

SAMPLE ITEM 3–3

Mr. Blake describes his son as being difficult to get *S T E M*
along with and concerned about what his friends *M*
think about him. How old is Mr. Blake's son?   **I T E M**

O
(1) 3 years old   DISTRACTOR   *P*
(2) 7 years old   DISTRACTOR   *T*
(3) 14 years old   CORRECT ANSWER   *I*
(4) 22 years old   DISTRACTOR   *O*
N
S

THE STEM

The stem is the initial part of a multiple-choice item. The purpose of the stem is to present a problem in a clear and concise manner. The stem should contain all the details necessary to answer the question. The stem of an item can be a complete sentence that asks a question. It can also be presented as an incomplete sentence that becomes a complete sentence when it is combined with one of the options in the item. In addition to sentence structure, a characteristic of a stem that must be considered is its polarity. The polarity of the stem can be formulated in either a positive or negative context. A *positive stem* asks the question in relation to what is true while a *negative stem* asks the question in relation to what is false.

The Stem That is a Complete Sentence

A complete sentence is a group of words that is capable of standing independently. When a stem is a complete sentence, it will pose a question and end with a question mark (?). It should clearly and concisely formulate a problem that could be answered before actually reading the options.

SAMPLE ITEM 3–4

What should be the first actions of the nurse when a fire alarm rings in a facility?

(1) Close all doors on the nursing unit

(2) Take an extinguisher to the fire scene

(3) Check the code chart to locate the fire

(4) Move patients laterally toward the stairs

SAMPLE ITEM 3–5

What is the most common reason why elderly patients become incontinent of urine?
(1) The aged tend to drink less fluid than younger patients.
(2) Their increase in weight places pressure on the bladder.
(3) They use incontinence to manipulate and control others.
(4) The muscles that control urination become weak.

SAMPLE ITEM 3–6

What part of the body requires special hygiene when a patient has a nasogastric feeding tube?
(1) Rectum
(2) Abdomen
(3) Oral cavity
(4) Perineal area

The Stem That is an Incomplete Sentence

When a stem is an incomplete sentence, it is a group of words that forms the beginning portion of a sentence. The sentence becomes complete when it is combined with one of the options in the item. Some tests will have a period at the completion of each option and others will not. Whether there is a period or not, each option should complete the sentence with grammatical accuracy. However, the answer is the only option that correctly completes the sentence in relation to the informational content. When reading a stem that is an incomplete sentence, it is usually necessary to read the options before the question can be answered.

SAMPLE ITEM 3–7

To best understand what a patient is saying, the nurse should:
(1) Demonstrate interest
(2) Listen carefully
(3) Remain silent
(4) Employ touch

SAMPLE ITEM 3–8

Patients should not be permitted to smoke in bed because it could:

(1) Result in a fire

(2) Upset the roommate

(3) Precipitate lung cancer

(4) Trigger the smoke alarm

SAMPLE ITEM 3–9

When assisting a patient with dementia to groom her hair, the nurse should:

(1) Set time aside for a long teaching session

(2) Offer constant support and encouragement

(3) Alternate using a brush and a comb

(4) Teach her how to braid her hair

The Stem With Positive Polarity

The stem with positive polarity is concerned with truth. It asks the question with a positive statement. The correct answer is accurately related to the statement. It is in accord with a fact or principle, or it is an action that should be implemented. A positively worded stem attempts to determine if you are able to understand, apply, or differentiate correct information.

SAMPLE ITEM 3–10

An elderly patient who is dying starts to cry and says, "I was always concerned about myself first and I hurt many people during my life." The nurse recognizes that the underlying feeling being expressed by the patient is:

(1) Ambivalence

(2) Sadness

(3) Guilt

(4) Anger

SAMPLE ITEM 3–11

Which of the following interventions most accurately supports the concept of informed consent?
(1) Obtaining the patient's signature
(2) Explaining what is being done and why
(3) Involving the family in the teaching plan
(4) Teaching preoperative deep breathing and coughing

SAMPLE ITEM 3–12

A patient appears to be asleep but does not react when his name is called. The nurse should:
(1) Inform the charge nurse immediately.
(2) Tell the patient, "Squeeze my hand."
(3) Gently touch the patient and softly call his name.
(4) Loudly call the patient's name and say, "Wake up."

The Stem With Negative Polarity

The stem with negative polarity is concerned with what is false. It asks the question with a negative statement. The stem usually incorporates words such as "except," "not," or "never." These words are obvious. However, sometimes the words that are used are more obscure, for example, "contraindicated," "unacceptable," "least," and "avoid." When a negative term is used it may be emphasized by an underline (except), italics (*least*), dark type (**not**), or capitals (NEVER). A negatively worded stem strives to ascertain if you can specify exceptions, detect errors, or identify interventions that are unacceptable or contraindicated. NCLEX-RN does not emphasize the negative word when used in a stem, and many schools do not have questions with negative polarity. However, this information has been included in the event that you may be challenged by questions with negative polarity.

SAMPLE ITEM 3–13

On what part of the body should the nurse avoid using soap when administering a bath to a patient on bed rest?
(1) Eyes
(2) Back
(3) Under the breasts
(4) Glans of the penis

SAMPLE ITEM 3–14

Range-of-motion exercises should NOT be done:
(1) For comatose patients
(2) On limbs that are paralyzed
(3) Beyond the point of resistance
(4) For patients with chronic joint disease

SAMPLE ITEM 3–15

When teaching the patient about promoting personal energy, the suggestion that would be **least** therapeutic would be:
(1) Eat breakfast every day
(2) Exercise three times a week
(3) Get adequate sleep each night
(4) Drink a cup of coffee each morning

SAMPLE ITEM 3–16

What position would be *contraindicated* for the patient who has dyspnea?
(1) Supine
(2) Contour
(3) Fowler's
(4) Orthopneic

SAMPLE ITEM 3–17

During a bed bath it would be unacceptable for the nurse to:
(1) Uncover the area being washed
(2) Wash from the rectum toward the pubis
(3) Use long firm strokes toward the heart
(4) Remove the top sheets and use a blanket

THE OPTIONS

All of the possible answers offered within an item are called "options." One of the options is the best response and is therefore the correct answer. The other options are incorrect and distract you from selecting the correct answer. These options are called "distractors." An item must have a minimum of three options to be considered a multiple-choice item, but the actual number varies among tests. The typical number of options is four or five responses which reduces the probability of guessing the correct answer while limiting the amount of reading to a sensible level. Options are usually listed by number (1, 2, 3, and 4), lowercase letters (a, b, c, and d), or uppercase letters (A, B, C, and D). The grammatical presentation of options can appear in four different formats. An option can be a sentence, complete the sentence begun in the stem, be an incomplete sentence, or be a single word.

The Option That is a Sentence

A sentence is a unit of language that contains a stated or implied subject and verb. It is a statement that contains an entire thought and is autonomous. Options can appear as complete sentences. Some tests will have a period at the end of these options and others will not. Whether there is a period or not, each option should be grammatically correct. When the option is a verbal response, it should be grammatically correct and incorporate the appropriate punctuation such as quotation marks (" "), commas (,) exclamation point (!), question mark (?), or period (.).

SAMPLE ITEM 3–18

Before gathering the equipment for a procedure, what should the nurse do first?

(1) Raise the patient's bed to its highest position
(2) Pull the patient's curtain for privacy
(3) Position the patient for the procedure
(4) Explain the procedure to the patient

SAMPLE ITEM 3–19

A Catholic patient tells the nurse that before being hospitalized she went to Mass and received Communion every morning. What should the nurse do to meet this patient's spiritual needs?

(1) Make arrangements for her to receive Communion
(2) Encourage the patient to say her rosary every day
(3) Have a priest administer the Sacrament of the Sick
(4) Transfer her to a room with another Catholic patient

SAMPLE ITEM 3–20

Mr. Hunter is crying, and the only word the nurse understands is "wife." What should the nurse respond?

(1) "I'm sure that your wife is fine."
(2) "You are concerned about your wife?"
(3) "What did your wife do to upset you?"
(4) "Do you expect your wife to visit today?"

The Option That Completes the Sentence Begun in the Stem

When the option completes the sentence begun in the stem, the stem and the option together should form a sentence. Some tests will have correct punctuation at the end of these options and others will not. Whether there is a period or not, each option should complete the stem in a manner that is grammatically accurate.

SAMPLE ITEM 3–21

The primary etiology of obesity is a:
(1) Lack of balance in the variety of nutrients.
(2) Glandular disorder that prevents weight loss.
(3) Psychological problem that causes overeating.
(4) Caloric intake that exceeds metabolic needs.

SAMPLE ITEM 3–22

The nurse can best prevent the patient from getting a chill during a bed bath by:
(1) Rubbing briskly to cause vasodilation
(2) Exposing just the area being washed
(3) Giving a hot drink before the bath
(4) Pulling the curtain around the bed

SAMPLE ITEM 3–23

The nurse is to assist a patient with a bed bath; however, the patient has just returned from x-ray, is in pain, and refuses to bathe. The nurse should:
(1) Cancel the bath today
(2) Encourage a shower instead
(3) Delay the bath until later
(4) Give a partial bath quickly

The Option That is an Incomplete Sentence

When an option is an incomplete sentence, it will be a group of words that do not contain all the parts of speech (e.g., nouns, verbs, and adjectives) necessary to construct a complete sentence. The option that is an incomplete sentence is usually a phrase or group of related words. Although not a complete sentence, it conveys a unit of thought, an idea, or a concept.

SAMPLE ITEM 3-24

Which of the following interventions is associated with all types of isolation?

(1) Donning a mask
(2) Wearing a gown
(3) Washing the hands
(4) Keeping visitors out

SAMPLE ITEM 3-25

When should mouth care be administered to an unconscious patient?

(1) Whenever necessary
(2) Every 4 hours
(3) Once a shift
(4) Twice a day

SAMPLE ITEM 3-26

Which of the following actions by the nurse would help meet a patient's basic need for security and safety?

(1) Addressing the patient by name
(2) Explaining what is going to be done
(3) Accepting a patient's angry behavior
(4) Ensuring that the patient gets adequate nutrition

The Option That is a Word

A word is a series of letters that form a term. It is the most basic unit of language and is capable of communicating a message. The option that is a single word can be almost any part of speech (e.g., noun, pronoun, verb, or adverb) as long as it conveys information.

SAMPLE ITEM 3-27

Which of the following is a primary source for obtaining information related to the independent functions of a nurse?

(1) Chart
(2) Patient
(3) Physician
(4) Supervisor

SAMPLE ITEM 3–28

When grooming a patient's hair, the nurse needs a physician's order for which of the following conditions?

(1) Lice
(2) Matting
(3) Dryness
(4) Dandruff

SAMPLE ITEM 3–29

What approach should be used by the nurse caring for a patient who is grieving?

(1) Confronting
(2) Supporting
(3) Avoiding
(4) Limiting

SAMPLE ITEM 3–30

What is the nurse doing when formulating a nursing diagnosis?

(1) Planning
(2) Assessing
(3) Analyzing
(4) Implementing

SAMPLE ITEM 3–31

Which word best describes feelings associated with a child in Erikson's stage of autonomy versus shame and doubt?

(1) Hers
(2) Mine
(3) Theirs
(4) Nobody

ANSWERS AND RATIONALES FOR SAMPLE ITEMS IN CHAPTER 3

An asterisk (*) is in front of the rationale that explains the correct answer.

3–1   (1) Unsafe; if unwashed, the hands will contaminate anything that is touched.
   * (2) Before touching anything in a room, the hands should be washed to remove microorganisms.
     (3) Same as #1.
     (4) Same as #1.

3–2 * (1) The tube enters the nose, passes through the posterior nasopharynx and esophagus, and enters the stomach through the cardiac sphincter.
     (2) These are passages between the trachea and bronchioles and are part of the respiratory system.
     (3) This is a passage between the posterior nasopharynx and bronchi and is part of the respiratory system.
     (4) This is distal to the stomach and is the first portion of the small intestine; a nasogastric tube is designed to be advanced into the stomach, not the duodenum.

3–3   (1) Toddlers are concerned about themselves and their autonomy, not others.
     (2) School-age children are easy to get along with and are concerned about their performance and achieving.
   * (3) Adolescents are concerned about their identity, independence, and peer relationships; this causes tension between them and their parents.
     (4) Young adults are developing intimate relationships and becoming socially responsible.

3–4   (1) The location of the fire must be identified first to determine if the nurse's unit is the unit in danger.
     (2) To do this, the location of the fire must be identified first.
   * (3) The location of the fire will influence the nurse's next action.
     (4) Unsafe; patients need to be moved only if they are in danger.

3–5   (1) Incontinence is unrelated to fluid intake.
     (2) The elderly do not necessarily gain weight; many lose weight because of the loss of subcutaneous fat associated with aging; body weight does not influence incontinence.
     (3) Untrue; most elderly people want to be independent and in control of their bodily functions.
   * (4) Muscles, particularly the perineal muscles, tend to lose strength as people age.

3–6   (1) Special care is unnecessary; care provided during a routine bed bath is adequate.
     (2) Same as #1.
   * (3) A nasogastric tube feeding generally negates the need to chew; with lack of chewing, salivation declines which causes drying of the mucous membranes.
     (4) Same as #1.

3–7   (1) While this may indicate acceptance and encourage ventilation of feelings, it does nothing to promote understanding.
   * (2) This is important to pick up key words and identify emotional themes within the message.

(3) Same as #1.

(4) Touch is used to communicate a message, not receive, understand, or interpret a message from another.

3–8 * (1) Confused, weak, or lethargic patients may drop lighted cigarettes or ashes which can ignite bed linens.

(2) Although smoking can physically and emotionally disturb a roommate, safety is the priority.

(3) Although smoking may precipitate lung cancer, safety is the priority.

(4) Smoking will not trigger a fire alarm; considerable smoke and/or heat are needed to set off a fire alarm.

3–9 (1) People with dementia cannot concentrate long enough for a prolonged teaching session; learning occurs best with short frequent teaching sessions.

* (2) People with dementia become easily confused and need support and encouragement to stay focused and motivated.

(3) This would promote confusion; patients with dementia need consistency.

(4) Braiding the hair involves cognitive and psychomotor skills that the patient with dementia probably does not possess.

3–10 (1) Ambivalence would demonstrate two simultaneous conflicting feelings.

(2) Although the patient may be unhappy about past behaviors, it is the underlying feeling of guilt about hurting others that precipitated the patient's statement.

* (3) Guilt is a painful feeling of self-reproach resulting from the belief that one has done something wrong.

(4) Anger is a feeling of displeasure caused by opposition or mistreatment and is demonstrated by words or gestures in an effort to fight back at the cause of the feeling.

3–11 (1) Although obtaining the patient's signature is part of consent, the signature by itself does not imply that the patient understands.

* (2) The patient's knowledge and understanding of what is going to be done, why it is being done, and what the outcomes will be is what constitutes being informed prior to giving consent.

(3) Although this may be done, it is the patient who must sign the informed consent.

(4) Although this is part of preoperative teaching, it would be unnecessary if the patient did not consent to surgery.

3–12 (1) The nurse needs to assess the patient further before informing the charge nurse.

(2) The nurse must first get the patient's attention before giving a direction.

* (3) This is the first step to further assess this patient; touch and sound stimulate two senses; using the patient's name is individualizing care.

(4) Speaking loudly could frighten the patient; an additional sense should be stimulated because the patient previously has not responded to a verbal intervention.

3–13 * (1) Soaps usually contain sodium or potassium salts of fatty acids which are irritating and can injure the sensitive tissues of the eyes.

(2) This area needs soap and water to remove perspiration that collects on the skin.

(3) Body surface areas that touch are dark, warm, moist areas that must be washed with soap and water to limit the growth of microorganisms.

(4) This area needs soap and water to remove perspiration, urine, and smegma.

3–14   (1) ROM should be performed for unconscious patients because they are usually immobile and are at risk for developing contractures.

    (2) Paralyzed limbs must be moved through full ROM by the nurse to prevent loss of range secondary to inactivity.

    * (3) Resistance indicates that there is strain on the muscles or joints; continuing ROM beyond the point of resistance could cause injury.

    (4) People with chronic joint disease usually need gentle ROM to keep the joints mobile; ROM is usually avoided in acute episodes associated with joint disease.

3–15   (1) Food contains nutrients and calories which provide energy.

    (2) Exercise promotes muscle tone and energy.

    (3) Sleep is restful and restorative.

    * (4) Caffeine, although a stimulant, can be harmful to the body.

3–16   * (1) In this position the abdominal contents press against the diaphragm impeding expansion of the lungs.

    (2) This position is desirable because the abdominal contents drop by gravity permitting efficient contraction of the diaphragm and expansion of the thoracic cavity.

    (3) Same as #2.

    (4) Same as #2.

3–17   (1) Just the area being washed should be exposed to permit adequate bathing and inspection.

    * (2) Unsafe; this would contaminate the urinary meatus with microorganisms from the perianal area.

    (3) This is desirable because it promotes venous return.

    (4) This is desirable because it absorbs moisture, provides warmth, and promotes privacy.

3–18   (1) This could be frightening if the patient does not know why it is being done; this also would be unsafe.

    (2) Same as #1.

    (3) Same as #1.

    * (4) This meets the patient's right to know why and how care will be provided.

3–19   * (1) This meets the patient's spiritual needs and is easily accomplished in a hospital setting.

    (2) This focuses on a different ritual and denies the patient's concerns about missing Mass and not receiving Communion.

    (3) Same as #2.

    (4) The nurse, not other patients, must assist the patient to meet spiritual needs.

3–20   (1) This is false reassurance and draws a conclusion based on insufficient information.

    * (2) This response encourages further communication which is necessary to obtain more information about what is upsetting the patient.

    (3) This is a judgmental statement not based on fact.

    (4) This is not an open-ended question that allows the patient to express concerns; it focuses on one thought and may cut off further communication.

3–21   (1) This would result in malnutrition, not necessarily obesity; it could also result in weight loss.

     (2) Although glandular disorders, such as hypothyroidism may result in obesity, they are not the primary causes of obesity.

     (3) This is only one of many factors that influence overeating; it is not the primary etiology of obesity.

* (4) If more calories are ingested than the body requires for energy, then they will be converted to adipose tissue which causes weight gain.

3–22   (1) Vasodilation promotes heat loss.

* (2) This limits evaporation of fluids on the skin and radiation of heat from the body which prevent a chill.

     (3) This will not prevent a chill.

     (4) While this may prevent drafts, it will not prevent a chill from the environmental temperature, excessive exposure, or evaporation of water from the skin.

3–23   (1) This may eventually be done, but the bath should be delayed first.

     (2) This ignores the patient's right to refuse care and the fact that the patient is in pain.

* (3) This accepts the patient's present refusal to bathe; rest and pain reduction may make the patient more amenable to hygiene later in the day.

     (4) Same as #2.

3–24   (1) A mask is worn for respiratory and strict isolation.

     (2) A gown is worn for strict isolation or if there is a potential for exposure to contaminated material.

* (3) This is required prior to and following care and is associated with all types of isolation.

     (4) Visitors are permitted in isolation after they have been taught how to maintain medical asepsis.

3–25 * (1) Unconscious patients usually have dry mucous membranes of the oral cavity because they frequently breathe through the mouth, are not drinking fluids, and may be receiving oxygen; oral hygiene is required whenever necessary, which is at least every 2 hours.

     (2) This is too long; drying, sordes, and lesions of the mucous membranes can occur.

     (3) Same as #2.

     (4) Same as #2.

3–26   (1) This meets the patient's need for self-esteem.

* (2) Knowing what will happen and why provides for security needs; it is also a patient's right; the unknown can be frightening.

     (3) Same as #1.

     (4) This meets the basic physiological need for adequate nutrients for body processes.

3–27   (1) This is a secondary source; it also contains physicians' orders that are dependent functions of the nurse.

* (2) The primary and most important source for obtaining information referring to the patient is the patient; also the independent functions of the nurse include interventions that relate to human responses which are identified by direct contact with the patient.

      (3) This is a secondary source; when the nurse follows a physician's order, it is a dependent function of the nurse.

      (4) This is a secondary source; independent functions of the nurse can be performed independently of others.

3–28 * (1) Head lice (*Pediculus capitis*) requires a physician's order for a medicated shampoo such as Kwell; the patient must be isolated until the hair is treated twice with the medicated shampoo and the room and belongings disinfected.

      (2) This can be corrected by brushing from the ends of the hair progressively working upward toward the scalp; this does not require a physician's order.

      (3) This can be minimized by brushing the hair several times daily to spread the oil down the shaft of the hair; this does not require a physician's order.

      (4) This can be minimized by regular shampooing of the hair and scalp; brushing the scalp and hair improves scalp circulation which helps prevent dandruff.

3–29   (1) This could take away the patient's current coping mechanisms and leave the patient defenseless.

   * (2) A patient who is grieving is using defenses to deal with the crisis; these defenses should be supported.

     (3) This would abandon the patient; the nurse should be present to provide support.

     (4) Same as #1.

3–30   (1) A nursing diagnosis should be made during the analysis phase before planning nursing care because the interventions should be appropriate for the focus of concern.

     (2) Assessing collects the data which must occur before it can be analyzed and nursing diagnoses formulated.

   * (3) Data must be clustered and interpreted to identify human responses that indicate potential or actual health problems that can be treated by the nurse; statements that indicate actual or potential health problems treatable by the nurse are nursing diagnoses.

     (4) Implementation is putting the plan of care into action, which occurs after analysis and planning.

3–31   (1) This word is associated with others rather than the self or self-interests.

   * (2) Toddlers are developing a sense of autonomy and are discovering the difference between independence and dependence; they are concerned about themselves and their mastery over their environment.

     (3) Same as #1.

     (4) Same as #1.

4 The Nursing Process

Problem solving is a scientific process that provides a framework for identifying solutions to complex problems. It is a step-by-step process that utilizes a systematic approach. One might say that scientific problem solving is a "blueprint" that can be followed to identify and solve problems. The concept of problem solving is not exclusively used by nurses. It also is used by other professionals to problem solve within the context of their own job responsibilities. Nurses use the problem-solving process to identify human responses and to plan, implement, and evaluate nursing care. When scientific problem solving is utilized within the context of nursing, it is known as the nursing process. The *nursing process* contains five steps: assessment, analysis, planning, implementation, and evaluation.

Because the nursing process is the method of critical thinking used by nurses to meet patients' needs, items on nursing examinations are designed to test utilization of this process. Well-written test items are not haphazard. They are carefully designed to test your knowledge of a specific concept, skill, theory, and so on from the perspective of one of the five steps of the nursing process. When reading an item, being able to identify its place within the nursing process should contribute to your ability to recognize what the test item is asking. To do this, you must focus on the critical words within the item.

This chapter explores the five steps of the nursing process: assessment, analysis, planning, implementation, and evaluation. Sample items are presented to demonstrate item construction as they relate to each step. Critical words associated with each step of the nursing process are illustrated within the sample items. Attempt to identify variations of critical words within the sample items indicating activities associated with each step of the nursing process. Practice answering the questions. The correct answers and the rationales for all the options of the sample items are at the end of this chapter. The more understanding you have about the focus of the item you are reading, the better you will be at identifying what is being asked and the greater your chances of identifying the correct answer.

ASSESSMENT

In assessment, data must be accurately collected, verified, and communicated. Assessment items are designed to test your knowledge of information, theories, principles, and skills related to the assessment of the patient. It establishes the foundation upon which nurses base the subsequent steps in the nursing process. Assessment questions will ask you to:

- Obtain vital statistics
- Perform a physical assessment
- Collect specimens
- Identify patient adaptations that are objective and subjective
- Identify patient adaptations that are verbal and nonverbal
- Identify adaptations that are normal or abnormal
- Utilize various data collection methods
- Identify sources of data
- Verify critical findings
- Identify commonalities and differences in response to illness
- Communicate information about assessments to appropriate members of the health team

Critical words used within a test item that generally indicate that the item is focused on assessment include "inspect," "identify," "verify," "observe," "notify," "check," "inform," "question," "communicate," "verbal" and "nonverbal," "signs and symptoms," "observe," "sources," "perceptions," and "check and assess." Most testing errors occur in the assessment phase of the nursing process when options are selected that:

- Collect insufficient data
- Have data that are inaccurately collected
- Use unscientific methods of data collection
- Rely on a secondary source rather than the primary source, the patient
- Contain irrelevant data
- Fail to verify data
- Reflect bias or prejudice
- Fail to accurately communicate data

Collecting Data

Collecting data is the first part of assessment. The nurse collects data through specific *methods of data collection* such as performing a physical examination, interviewing, and reviewing records. A physical examination includes the assessment techniques of inspection, palpation, auscultation, and percussion. It includes obtaining the vital signs and recognizing normal and abnormal parameters of obtained values. Interviewing is used to collect data using a formal approach (e.g., obtaining a health history) or by an informal approach (e.g., exploring feelings while providing other nursing care). Review of records includes reports such as the results of laboratory test, diagnostic procedures, and assessments or consultations by other members of the health team.

SAMPLE ITEM 4–1

While making rounds, the nurse finds a patient on the floor in the hall. The initial response by the nurse should be to:

(1) Inspect the patient for injury

(2) Transfer the patient back to bed

(3) Move the patient to the closest chair

(4) Report the incident to the nursing supervisor

This item tests your ability to recognize that in an emergency situation the nurse must first assess the condition of the patient. This is a principle basic to any emergency response by a nurse. Moving a patient prior to an assessment could worsen any injury. This item demonstrates how a basic concept related to assessment can be tested.

SAMPLE ITEM 4–2

To avoid patient accidents, the nurse should:

(1) Assess the strength of a patient prior to activity

(2) Provide a cane for ambulating if the patient is weak

(3) Keep an overbed table in front of a sitting patient

(4) Utilize a vest restraint for a patient in a wheelchair

This item tests your ability to recognize the concept that the nurse must assess a patient before implementing care. The three distractors are all concerned with implementing care. This question also tests your ability to recognize physical examination as a method of collecting data about the status of a patient.

SAMPLE ITEM 4–3

The nurse should identify that a patient is having difficulty when the respirations are:

(1) 16 per minute and deep

(2) 18 per minute and through the mouth

(3) 20 per minute and shallow

(4) 28 per minute and noisy

This item tests your ability to identify the option that reflects a respiratory rate and characteristic that is outside normal parameters. To successfully answer this question, the nurse needs to know the rate and characteristics of normal, as well as abnormal, respirations.

SAMPLE ITEM 4–4

When taking a rectal temperature, the nurse should always:
(1) Allow the patient to insert the thermometer
(2) Position the patient on the left side
(3) Use an electronic thermometer
(4) Lubricate the thermometer

Option 4 identifies what must be done (a critical element) to safely take a rectal temperature. The three distractors may or may not be done when obtaining a rectal temperature. Although this appears to be an implementation question because it involves an action, it is actually an assessment question because it is concerned with collecting data.

SAMPLE ITEM 4–5

When determining if a person's body weight is appropriate, it is important to assess the person's:
(1) Body height
(2) Daily intake
(3) Clothing size
(4) Food preferences

This item tests your ability to recognize that to calculate the patient's ideal body weight, the nurse must also know the patient's height. The ideal body weight is the measurement that reflects the range of weight that would be considered appropriate in relation to the patient's height. The ideal body weight is the measurement against which the patient's present weight is compared to determine if the patient is underweight or obese. Although the question does not address these concepts, the nurse must also know the patient's age and extent of bone structure.

Types of data collected when assessing a patient can be objective or subjective. *Objective data* are measurable assessments collected when the nurse uses sight, touch, smell, and hearing to acquire information. Examples of objective data include an excoriated perineal area, diaphoretic skin, ammonia odor to urine, rhonchi, and vital signs. *Subjective data* can be collected only when the patient shares feelings, perceptions, thoughts, and sensations about a health problem or concern. Examples of subjective data include patient statements about pain, shortness of breath, or feeling depressed.

to page 47

SAMPLE ITEM 4-6

The wife of a patient with painful terminal cancer says her husband is depressed. When talking with the patient, he states, "Life is not worth living. I'm going to kill myself." The nurse recognizes that the patient's statement is:

(1) Primary data
(2) Objective data
(3) Secondary data
(4) Subjective data

This item tests your ability to differentiate the types of data collected during the assessment phase of the nursing process. The nurse should know the type of data collected for the purpose of future clustering and determining significance. Any information that a patient shares regarding feelings, thoughts, and concerns are subjective. This question also incorporates the concept that the patient is the primary source.

Data can be gathered not only by different methods but also from different sources. *Sources of data* available to the nurse include those that are primary, secondary, or tertiary. There is only one *primary source,* the patient. The nurse must be able to recognize significant signs and symptoms exhibited or verbalized by the patient and be able to determine the patient's ability to provide for one's own activities of daily living. The patient is the most valuable source because the data that are collected are most current and specific to the patient. A *secondary source* produces information from someplace other than the patient. A family member is a secondary source who can contribute information about the patient's likes and dislikes, ethnic and cultural background, similarities and differences in behavior, and functioning before and during the health problem. The patient's chart is another example of a secondary source. It is a legal document comprising information that concerns the patient's physical, psychosocial, religious, and economic history and documents the patient's physical and emotional adaptations. Controversy surrounds the labeling of diagnostic test results in a chart as being either primary or secondary sources. Although the chart itself is a secondary source, diagnostic test results are direct objective measurements of the patient's status and therefore are considered by some healthcare providers to be a primary source. The nurse must remember that the information in a chart is history and does not reflect the current status of the patient because the patient is dynamic and constantly changing. The patient's immediate environment should also be considered a secondary source of data. Nurses need to assess the immediate environment to establish a database upon which to base decisions regarding the need for planning interventions to protect a patient's safety. Secondary sources are valuable for gathering supplementary information about a patient. A *tertiary source* provides information from outside the specific patient's frame of reference. Examples of tertiary sources include textbooks, the nurse's experience, and accepted commonalities among patients with similar adaptations. Included under tertiary sources are the nurse's or other staff members' responses to the patient, the patient's significant others, and other health team members.

SAMPLE ITEM 4–7

The nurse asks a patient's wife specific questions about the patient's health complaints prior to admission. When collecting this information, the nurse is seeking information from a:

(1) Primary source
(2) Tertiary source
(3) Secondary source
(4) Subjective source

This item tests your ability to recognize that a family member is a secondary source of information. Secondary sources provide information that is supplemental to the primary information collected from the patient.

Collected data can be verbal or nonverbal. *Verbal data* are collected via the spoken word. For example, statements to the nurse by the patient are verbal data. *Nonverbal data* are collected via transmission of a message without words. Crying, a fearful facial expression, the appearance of the patient, and gestures are all examples of nonverbal data.

SAMPLE ITEM 4–8

An example of nonverbal communication is:

(1) A letter
(2) Holding hands
(3) Noise in the room
(4) A telephone message

This item tests your ability to recognize that holding hands is a form of nonverbal communication. Nonverbal communication does not use words. Touch, gestures, posture, and facial expressions are examples of nonverbal communication.

When assessing and collecting data, nurses should use both inductive and deductive reasoning. *Deductive reasoning* moves from the general to the specific. For example, the nurse can use deductive reasoning when collecting data about a patient who has a body cast. If it is accepted that patients in a body cast generally are at risk for altered skin integrity, then the nurse should recognize the need to assess this specific patient's skin for early signs of impaired skin integrity. *Inductive reasoning* moves from the specific to the general. For example, the nurse uses inductive reasoning when collecting data related to a specific postoperative patient's weak thready pulse. The nurse is aware that a weak thready pulse can indicate postoperative hemorrhage. From this specific assessment the nurse recognizes the need to further assess for additional general signs of hemorrhage such as a drop in blood pressure, increased respirations, and cold clammy skin. Effective inductive and deductive reasoning are based on a strong theoretical foundation of knowledge that is drawn upon when collecting data.

SAMPLE ITEM 4–9

A patient is drinking 3000 ml of fluid a day. When assessing the patient's urine, the nurse can expect the urine to be:

(1) Dark straw colored

(2) Straw colored

(3) Light amber

(4) Dark amber

This item tests your ability to use deductive reasoning to identify an expected common response to fluid intake of 3000 ml a day. It is a known fact that the more fluid a person drinks, the lighter the color of the urine. Straw colored is the only option that is within normal parameters.

Verifying Data

Once data are collected, they must be verified. *Verifying data* is the confirming of information by collecting additional data, questioning orders, obtaining judgments and/or conclusions from other team members when appropriate, and by collecting data oneself rather than relying on technology. Verifying data ensures authenticity and accuracy. For example, when a vital statistic is outside the normal range or is a measurement that is unexpected, the nurse must substantiate the results by collecting the data again and/or collecting additional data to supplement the original information.

SAMPLE ITEM 4–10

The nurse takes the patient's blood pressure and records a diastolic pressure of 120. The nurse should first:

(1) Take the other vital signs

(2) Retake the blood pressure

(3) Notify the charge nurse

(4) Notify the physician

This item tests your ability to recognize that the nurse needs to verify data when they are unexpected or outside normal parameters. The first action by the nurse should be to retake the blood pressure after waiting a minute. The nurse may have made an error when taking the blood pressure. Once the blood pressure is verified as being outside normal parameters, then the nurse should take the other vital signs and notify the physician of the results.

Communicating Information about Assessments

The last component of assessment includes the nurse's ability to communicate information obtained from assessment activities. Sharing vital information about a patient is essential if members of the health team are to be alerted to the most current status of the patient. Communication methods vary (e.g., progress notes, verbal notification, flow sheets); however, they all share the need to be accurate, concise, thorough, current, organized, and confidential.

SAMPLE ITEM 4–11

After verifying that the patient's vital signs were unexpectedly outside normal parameters, the nurse should:

(1) Initiate a code

(2) Notify the physician

(3) Inform the supervisor

(4) Reassess the vital signs in 30 minutes

     This item tests your ability to recognize that once a nurse identifies that a patient's vital signs are significantly abnormal, the physician should be immediately notified. Communicating data to appropriate health team members is a component of the assessment process.

ANALYSIS

Analysis is the second step of the nursing process and is the most difficult component. Analysis requires the interpretation of data, collection of additional data, identification and communication of nursing diagnoses, and assurance that the patient's health care needs are appropriately met. To be interpreted, data must be validated, clustered, and its significance determined before making a nursing diagnosis that identifies the patient's nursing problem. The nursing diagnosis is part of the nursing care plan. To analyze data, you will need to have a strong foundation in scientific principles related to nursing theory, social sciences, and physical sciences, and you will need to know the commonalities and differences in patients' responses to various stresses. You will need to use deductive and inductive reasoning to apply your knowledge and experience when answering analysis items. Analysis questions will ask you to:

- Cluster data
- Identify clustered data as meaningful
- Validate data
- Interpret validated and clustered data
- Identify when additional data are necessary to validate clustered data
- Identify nursing diagnoses
- Communicate nursing diagnoses to others
- Ensure that the patient's health care needs can be appropriately met

Critical words used within a test item that generally indicate that the item is focused on analysis include "valid," "organize," "categorize," "cluster," "reexamine," "pattern," "formulate," "nursing diagnosis," "reflect," "relate," "problem," "interpret," "contribute," "relevant," "decision," "significant," "deduction," "statement," and "analysis." See if you can identify variations of these critical words indicating analysis activities in the sample items in this chapter. Testing errors occur in the analysis phase of the nursing process when options are selected that:

- Cluster data prematurely
- Omit data
- Make a nursing diagnosis before all significant data have been clustered
- Force the nursing diagnosis to fit the signs and symptoms collected

Interpretation of Data

Interpretation of data is a critical step in the process of analysis. It is related to the nurse's ability to validate data, cluster data, determine significance of clustered data, and come to a conclusion. In analysis the nurse validates data to determine their significance. Information is more meaningful when its relationship to other data is established. Clustering enables the nurse to organize data; eliminate that which is insignificant, irrelevant, and redundant; and reduce the remaining data into manageable categories. Data must first be organized into general categories such as physical, sociocultural, and psychological. Once organized into general categories, they are clustered specifically based on the health care needs of the patient. To cluster data, the nurse needs to group related information. To do this effectively, the nurse must refer to theoretical knowledge and scientific principles, the database that identifies the patient's specific adaptation to stress, and the practice of clinical judgment. This process depends on a combination of intellectual skills. The nurse uses deductive and inductive reasoning drawing from knowledge of commonalities and differences. These same intellectual skills also are used to determine significance of clustered data. "Significance" in this context refers to some consequence, importance, implication, or gravity connected to the cluster as it relates to the patient's health problem. Data can be overt and easy to cluster or covert and difficult to cluster. Some data are easily clustered because the information collected is clearly related to only one system of the body. Other data are more difficult to cluster because the patient's adaptations may involve a variety of systems of the body. At first the facts collected may not appear to be related. However, with a thorough analysis the nurse recognizes that the data are interrelated.

to page 52

SAMPLE ITEM 4–12

The patient had a stroke that left her paralyzed on the right side. When clustering data, the nurse grouped the following data together: drooling of saliva, slurred speech, and left-sided weakness. To complete this cluster of data, which of the following would be most significant?

(1) Expressive aphasia

(2) Difficulty swallowing

(3) Inability to perform ADLs

(4) Incontinent of urine and stool

This item tests your ability to recognize a cluster of data that indicates that a patient is at risk for aspiration. Oxygenation is a basic physiological need. A patient who is drooling saliva, has slurred speech, has left-sided weakness, and has difficulty swallowing would be at serious risk for aspiration of material into the respiratory tract. While the other options are all problems that must be addressed by the nurse, they are not data related to oxygenation and have no significance to this specific cluster.

SAMPLE ITEM 4–13

Decubitus ulcers are most often associated with patients who:

(1) Are immobilized

(2) Have psychiatric diagnoses

(3) Experience respiratory distress

(4) Need close supervision for safety

This item tests your ability to recognize the relationship between immobility and the formation of decubitus ulcers. It is designed to test your knowledge of the need for cellular oxygenation; how immobility can cause pressure; and how pressure can interfere with the body's ability to oxygenate local cellular tissue.

Once significance is determined, a deduction is made regarding the clustered data. A *deduction* is defined as forming a conclusion from clustered data. Deductions are inferred from nursing theory, collected data unique to the patient, accepted general theories, and the physical and social sciences. Deductive reasoning is used to accomplish this task. Deductive reasoning moves from the general to the specific.

to page 53

SAMPLE ITEM 4–14

A patient has anorexia and insomnia and has lost interest in activities of daily living. This behavior is reflective of feelings related to:

(1) Anger
(2) Denial
(3) Depression
(4) Acceptance

This item tests your ability to make a deduction based on a cluster of data. The word "reflective" in the stem cues you to the fact that this is an analysis question. You need to draw from your knowledge of commonalities of human behavior and use deductive reasoning to arrive at the conclusion that the patient is probably depressed.

SAMPLE ITEM 4–15

Mr. Evans is debilitated and unsteady on his feet. He insists on walking to the bathroom by himself without calling for assistance. This behavior reflects a need to be:

(1) Alone
(2) Accepted
(3) Independent
(4) Manipulative

This item also tests your ability to make a deduction based on a cluster of data. To answer this question, you must analyze and interpret the information in the stem and come to a conclusion. Your knowledge of human behavior and use of deductive reasoning should enable you to select the correct answer.

Collection of Additional Data

Once significance is determined but before making a final deduction, additional data collection might be indicated to provide more information to support the deduction. This is done to establish and ensure the relationship among the original data. The nurse continually reassesses the condition of the patient and the presence of needs, recognizing that the patient is dynamic and ever changing throughout all phases of the nursing process.

```
┌──────────────────────────────────────────────────┐
│ ██████████████████████████████████████████████   │
│    SAMPLE ITEM 4–16                               │
│ ██████████████████████████████████████████████   │
│                                                    │
│  The nurse assesses that a postoperative patient   │
│  is exhibiting a decreased blood pressure and      │
│  weak thready pulse. The nurse should reassess     │
│  the patient for additional signs of:              │
│  (1) Hemorrhage                                    │
│  (2) Infection                                     │
│  (3) Anxiety                                       │
│  (4) Pain                                          │
│                                                    │
│       This item is designed to test your ability   │
│  to recognize that the nurse needs to reassess a   │
│  patient for additional data to reinforce the      │
│  proposed deduction. Hypotension and weak          │
│  thready pulse are related to a decreased blood    │
│  volume which is associated with postoperative     │
│  hemorrhage.                                       │
└──────────────────────────────────────────────────┘
```

Identifying and Communicating Nursing Diagnoses

Taking a deduction and converting it into a diagnostic statement is called making a nursing diagnosis. It moves from a general statement of a problem (a deduction) into a specific statement (a nursing diagnosis). A *nursing diagnosis* is a statement of a specific health problem that a nurse is legally permitted to treat. The diagnostic statement should include the problem and the factors that contribute to the development of the problem. It is important to include the contributing factors because while two patients may have the same problem, it can be caused by different stresses. This concept is important because the nature of the contributing factors drives the choice of interventions being planned. For example, two patients have altered skin integrity. However, one patient's skin problem is related to incontinence and edema, and the other patient's skin problem is related to immobility and pressure. The interventions may be very different because the factors contributing to the problem are different. This will be discussed in more detail in the section in this chapter titled "Planning." Nurses use the taxonomy of nursing diagnoses developed by the North American Nursing Diagnosis Association (NANDA) as a blueprint. This taxonomy provides for classifying nursing problems, standardizing language, facilitating communication, and focusing on an individualized approach to identifying and meeting a patient's nursing needs. The following are examples of *nursing diagnoses:*

- High risk for impaired skin integrity related to incontinence
- Feeding self-care deficit related to bilateral arm casts
- Ineffective airway clearance related to excessive secretions

Nurses need to communicate nursing diagnoses to other nurses via the *nursing care plan* (NCP). The NCP includes the nursing diagnosis, expected outcomes, and planned nursing interventions. The section of this chapter titled "Planning" will discuss outcomes and planned nursing interventions in more detail.

SAMPLE ITEM 4–17

The patient has suffered a stroke, has left-sided hemiparesis, and is incontinent. Which of the following is an appropriately worded nursing diagnosis for this patient?

(1) The patient has a need to maintain skin integrity.

(2) The patient will be clean and dry and will receive range-of-motion exercises every 4 hours.

(3) The patient has a stroke evidenced by hemiparesis and incontinence secondary to a cerebral vascular accident.

(4) The patient is at high risk for impaired skin integrity related to left-sided hemiparesis and incontinence secondary to a stroke.

This item tests your ability to recognize language used by the North American Nursing Diagnosis Association (NANDA) taxonomy. Use of NANDA-approved terminology is a current nursing standard of practice. To answer this item correctly, you must be able to recognize the differences among a patient need, an expected outcome, a nursing intervention, and a properly stated nursing diagnosis as it relates to a cluster of data.

Ensuring That Patients' Health Care Needs Are Appropriately Met

The health team has a responsibility to ensure the public that health care needs will be appropriately met. During the analysis phase of the nursing process, the nurse may identify that the patient's health care needs cannot be met by the nurse providing the care because the nurse is unprepared, the nurse is inexperienced in caring for a patient with a particular problem, or there is inadequate staffing. If the nurse perceives a risk to patient safety, the nurse is obligated to take an action that will ensure that appropriate care will be provided. This might necessitate rearranging the assignment with other nurses on the unit, or it may require intervention by the nurse supervisor. Once the nurse embarks on a duty of care, the nurse is obligated to provide a standard of care defined by the nurse practice act in the state in which the nurse works.

to page 56

```
SAMPLE ITEM 4–18

The night charge nurse arrives on duty and discovers that
several staff members have just called in sick. The nurse's
most appropriate response would be to:
(1) Inform the supervisor and ask for additional staff
(2) Identify which patients need care and assign staff
    accordingly
(3) Stay, but refuse to accept responsibility for the standard
    of care delivered on the unit
(4) Explain to patients that when the unit is short staffed,
    only essential care can be provided

    This item tests your ability to recognize your responsi-
bility to ensure that patients' needs are appropriately met.
Once the nurse perceives a risk to patient safety, the nurse
is obligated to take action that will ensure that appropriate
care will be provided.
```

PLANNING

Planning is the third step of the nursing process. It involves setting goals, establishing priorities, identifying expected outcomes, identifying interventions designed to achieve goals and outcomes, modifying the plan as necessary, and collaborating with other health team members to ensure that care is coordinated. Goals, outcomes, and identified interventions are formulated in response to the nursing diagnoses that were identified in the previous step (analysis) of the nursing process. The nursing diagnoses, goals, outcomes, and identified interventions make up the *nursing care plan* (NCP). It is the nursing care plan that outlines the nursing care for each patient. To plan care, you will need to have a strong foundation of scientific theory; know the commonalities and differences in response to nursing interventions; and know the theories related to establishing priority of needs. You will need to use deductive reasoning to apply your knowledge and clinical experience when answering planning questions. Planning items will ask you to:

- Set goals
- Establish priorities
- Plan appropriate interventions
- Involve the patient in the planning process
- Anticipate patient needs
- Recognize the need to collaborate with others
- Recognize that plans must be flexible and modified based on changing patient needs
- Recognize the need to coordinate planned care with other disciplines
- Establish expected outcomes against which results of care can be compared for the purpose of evaluation

Critical words used within a test item that generally indicate that the item is focused on planning include "achieve," "desired," "plan," "effective," "desired result," "goal," "priority," "develop," "formulate," "establish," "design," "prevent," "strategy," "select," "determine," "anticipate," "modify," "collaborate," "arrange," "coordinate," "expect," and "outcome." See if you can identify variations of these critical words indicating planning activities in the sample items in this chapter. Testing errors occur during the planning phase when options are selected that:

- Do not include the patient in setting goals and priorities
- Are inappropriate goals
- Misidentify priorities
- Reflect outcomes that are unrealistic and unmeasurable
- Reflect planned interventions that are inappropriate or incomplete
- Fail to include family members and significant others when appropriate
- Reflect poorly written care plans
- Fail to coordinate and collaborate with other health team members

The planning component of the nursing process generates a statement of goals, expected outcomes, and interventions that are planned to meet these goals and outcomes. This plan, called the nursing care plan, becomes the blueprint for nursing interventions that is dictated by the patient's individual needs and preferences.

Identifying Goals

Goals are general statements that direct nursing interventions, provide broad parameters for measuring results, and stimulate motivation. Goals can be long-term or short-term. A *long-term goal* is one that will take time to achieve (weeks to months). A long-term goal for a patient who has a stroke might be, "Mr. Brown will provide for his own activities of daily living by discharge." A *short-term goal* is one that can be achieved relatively quickly (usually within a week or two). A short-term goal might say, "Mr. Brown will wash his hands and face daily." Eventually the goal is further developed to become the expected outcome. Projecting expected outcomes will be discussed in more detail later in this chapter.

to page 58

SAMPLE ITEM 4–19

The nurse is caring for a patient with a temporary colostomy. Which of the following would be a realistic short-term goal for this patient?

(1) The patient will have regular bowel elimination.

(2) The patient's bowel will function within 2 days.

(3) The patient's skin will remain intact around the stoma.

(4) The patient will be at high risk for impaired skin integrity.

This item tests your ability to recognize a short-term goal. To answer this question, you need to know commonalities related to caring for a patient with a temporary colostomy and be able to recognize the differences among short- and long-term goals, a nursing diagnosis, and an outcome statement.

Setting Priorities

Setting priorities is an important step in the planning process. Once nursing diagnoses and goals are identified, they must be ranked in order of importance. Maslow's hierarchy of needs is helpful in establishing priorities. Basic physiological needs are ranked first, with the need for safety and security, belonging and love, self-esteem, and self-actualization following in rank order. It is important, however, to recognize that at one point in time any one of Maslow's needs may take priority depending upon the needs of the individual patient. Obviously if someone is choking on food, clearing the airway would take priority. However, there are times when the emergency or immediate need of the patient is in the psychological dimension. The nurse must be aware of the patient's perceptions and perspective when setting priorities because patients are the center of the health team. When possible, the patient should always be involved in setting priorities.

to page 59

SAMPLE ITEM 4-20

A patient has just returned from surgery with an IV and does not have a gag reflex. Which of the following planned interventions takes priority?

(1) Ensure correct placement of the oral airway

(2) Observe the dressing for drainage

(3) Check for IV infiltration

(4) Monitor vital signs

This item tests your ability to prioritize care. All of these planned interventions are important. However, oxygenation is essential to sustain life and therefore maintaining a patent airway is the priority.

Identifying Interventions

After priorities are established, a plan for nursing action must be formulated. To appropriately plan, the nurse must rely on scientific knowledge, clinical judgment, and knowledge about the patient and use the reasoning process. Relying on this background, the nurse determines what nursing measures would be most effective in assisting the patient to achieve a goal or outcome. For example, when caring for a patient with a decubitus ulcer, the nurse reasons, "If I turn and reposition the patient and massage around the area with lotion every 2 hours, then circulation will increase and healing will be promoted." When planning care, the nurse must know the rationales for nursing interventions so that the interventions selected are the most appropriate for the patient care situation.

SAMPLE ITEM 4-21

The most effective way to prevent the spread of the flu in a hospital is by:

(1) Limiting the spread of microorganisms

(2) Utilizing strict isolation precautions

(3) Administering antibiotics to sick patients

(4) Keeping the patient's windows closed during the winter

This item tests your ability to recognize that planning to limit the spread of microorganisms can prevent the spread of infection. This question focuses on a general concept applicable to all patients because it involves planning a variety of interventions that can protect many patients.

SAMPLE ITEM 4–22

Mr. Koller is on bed rest, and his bed needs a complete change of linen. The nurse should plan to:
(1) Make an occupied bed
(2) Raise him with a mechanical lift
(3) Change the draw sheet and top sheet
(4) Transfer him to a chair during the linen change

    This item tests your ability to recognize the needs of a patient on bed rest. The word "plan" used in the stem is an obvious clue that this is a planning question.

SAMPLE ITEM 4–23

An occupied bed must be made for a patient who is:
(1) Obese
(2) Immobile
(3) In a cast
(4) On bed rest

    This item is similar to Sample Item 4–22; however, the content of the stem and the correct option are reversed. This item is more difficulty to identify as a planning item because the word "plan" is not in the stem.

Projecting Expected Outcomes

Expected outcomes are the changes in the patient's condition that are expected in response to care given. Expected outcomes are derived from goal statements, but they are more specific because they describe the behavior or data that should be demonstrated once the goal is achieved. Expected outcomes are the benchmarks against which the actual outcomes are compared to determine the effectiveness of the interventions provided. To be meaningful, they must be patient centered, specific, realistic, measurable, and within a certain time frame. The actual process of comparing actual outcomes with expected outcomes occurs in the evaluation phase, which is the next step in the nursing process. Examples of outcomes are, "The patient brushes her teeth after every meal," "The patient states a reduction in anxiety in one week," and "The patient's diastolic blood pressure is below 90 mm Hg by discharge." Sometimes the nurse may state goals and outcomes together. For example, "The patient will continuously maintain an effective airway clearance as evidenced by expectoration of sputum, clear lung fields, and noiseless breathing." The first part of the statement is the goal, and what follows *as evidenced by* are the expected outcomes. The first part of the statement is more general, and the second part is more specific.

SAMPLE ITEM 4–24

A nurse is caring for a patient experiencing anorexia and vomiting. Which of the following would be a statement of an expected outcome?

(1) The patient will maintain a weight of 160 pounds in the next 14 days.

(2) The patient has altered nutrition less than body requirements.

(3) The patient's privacy will be maintained when providing patient care.

(4) The patient's mouth will be cleaned every 4 hours.

This item tests your ability to recognize a statement that reflects an expected outcome. To answer this question, you need to know commonalities of caring for a patient with anorexia and vomiting. You also need to recognize the differences among a goal, an expected outcome, a nursing diagnosis, and a nursing intervention.

Modifying the Plan of Care As Needed

Planning generally takes place prior to care being given. However, patient needs sometimes change while the nurse is in the process of implementing care, and a plan must be immediately modified. It is important to recognize that plans of care are not set in stone but are modified in response to the changing needs of the patient. Because a patient's needs are dynamic, the NCP is also dynamic. It must be continually changed to be kept current, substituting new nursing diagnoses, goals, and planned interventions as indicated by the patient's changing needs.

to page 62

```
SAMPLE ITEM 4–25
```

A patient is receiving oxygen by nasal cannula. After morning care the patient experiences dyspnea and complains of feeling tired. When planning for this patient's bath the next day, the nurse should:

(1) Give a complete bath as quickly as possible

(2) Bathe only those body parts that are necessary

(3) Arrange for several rest periods during morning care

(4) Continue with the same plan because dyspnea is unavoidable

This item tests your ability to recognize the need to modify a plan of care based on new data. The words "planning" in the stem and "arrange" in the correct answer are obvious clues that this is a planning question.

Collaborating with Other Health Team Members

Another component of planning is consultation and collaboration with other health team members to brainstorm, seek additional input, and delegate and coordinate the delivery of health services. The nurse is responsible for coordinating the members of the nursing team as well as the entire health team. The nurse manages the members of the nursing team by appropriately delegating and supervising nursing interventions. The plan also identifies and coordinates the services of other departments within the hospital. The nurse is responsible for ensuring that services such as laboratory tests, radiological studies, and physical therapy are performed within the context of the patient's physical and emotional abilities. For example, the nurse may arrange for a patient to go to physical therapy in the morning before the patient tires, or the nurse may consult with the dietitian for help with designing a menu that incorporates a patient's preferences. Effective planning contributes to the delivery of patient care that has continuity and is patient centered, coordinated, and individualized.

to page 63

SAMPLE ITEM 4–26

The nurse is caring for a patient with a large decubitus ulcer that has not responded to common nursing interventions. To best deal with this problem, the nurse should consult with the:

(1) Plastic surgeon

(2) Physical therapist

(3) Attending physician

(4) Clinical nurse specialist

This item is designed to test your ability to recognize that planning nursing care may require the nurse to seek the expertise of a specialist. A clinical nurse specialist is educated and prepared to provide expert advice and lend problem-solving and educational skills to seek solutions to difficult clinical nursing problems. While the nurse consults with health team members of other disciplines for various reasons, the nurse should consult with a clinical nurse specialist or other resources in nursing for assistance with solving nursing problems.

IMPLEMENTATION

Implementation is the step of the nursing process whereby planned actions are initiated and completed. It includes tasks such as organizing and managing planned care; providing total or partial assistance with activities of daily living (ADL); counseling and teaching the patient and significant others; providing planned care; supervising, coordinating, and evaluating the process of the delivery of care by the nursing staff (this does not include the actual delegation of care that occurs in planning or the evaluation of the patient's response to care which occurs in evaluation); and recording and sharing data related to care implemented.

To implement safe nursing care designed to achieve goals and expected outcomes, the nurse must understand and follow the implementation process. In addition, the nurse must have knowledge of scientific rationales for nursing procedures; psychomotor skills to implement procedures safely, and the ability to utilize different strategies to effectively implement nursing care. Implementation items will ask you to:

- Recognize steps in the implementation process
- Identify independent, dependent, and interdependent actions of the nurse
- Implement a procedure or treatment
- Identify and respond to common or uncommon outcomes in response to interventions
- Identify or respond to life-threatening or adverse events
- Prepare a patient for a procedure, treatment, or surgery
- Choose an approach that is most appropriate when implementing care
- Identify safe or unsafe practice

- Rationalize a step in a procedure
- Identify or utilize concepts related to teaching
- Identify or utilize concepts related to counseling
- Identify or utilize principles related to motivation and therapeutic communication
- Recognize the relationship between a procedure and an expected outcome
- Identify when an intervention must be modified in response to a change in the patients's condition
- Identify when additional assistance is required to provide safe care
- Recognize the nurse's responsibility associated with supervising and evaluating care delivered by those to whom interventions have been delegated
- Recognize how and when to document or report care given along with the patient's response

Critical words used within a test item that generally indicate that the item is focused on implementation include "dependent," "independent," "intradependent," "change," "assist," "counsel," "teach," "give," "supervise," "perform," "method," "procedure," "treatment," "instruct," "strategy," "reassess," "facilitate," "provide," "inform," "refer," "technique," "motivate," "delegate," and "implement." See if you can identify variations of these critical words indicating implementation activities in the sample items. Testing errors occur during the implementation phase of the nursing process when options are selected that:

- Implement actions outside the definition of nursing practice
- Fail to identify or appropriately respond to an adverse or life-threatening situation
- Fail to reassess the patient
- Fail to modify interventions in response to the changing needs of the patient
- Fail to identify when additional assistance is required for the delivery of safe care
- Reflect a lack of knowledge to safely implement interventions
- Do not accurately document the patient's response to care given
- Fail to supervise and evaluate the delivery of delegated interventions

The Process of Implementation

Effective implementation of nursing care is based on:
- Reassessing the patient
- Reviewing and modifying the plan of care when indicated
- Identifying when additional help in either staff or resources is needed to safely implement the plan
- Implementing types of interventions
- Utilizing methods of intervention
- Communicating strategies verbally or in writing

The first three actions listed above have been discussed in detail in previous steps from the perspective of assessment, analysis, and planning. When considered from the perspective of intervention, the nurse must remember that the principles described in the preceding sections apply here as well. The concept to be internalized is that these actions are ongoing throughout the nursing process. The last three actions listed above are discussed next in more detail.

Types of Interventions

Interventions can be dependent, independent, or interdependent in nature. *Dependent interventions* are interventions that require a physician's order. Administering a medication, providing IV fluids, and inserting a nasogastric tube are examples of dependent interventions because they all require a physician's order. When implementing a dependent intervention, the nurse does not blindly follow the order but determines whether the order is correct or appropriate. A nurse who does not question and carries out an incorrect or inappropriate order is contributing to the initial error and will be held accountable. *Independent interventions* are those actions that a nurse is legally permitted to implement with no direction or supervision from others. Independent interventions do not require a physician's order. Tasks related to collecting data, providing assistance with ADLs, teaching regarding health, and counseling are in the realm of independent legal nursing practice. Encouraging coughing and deep breathing, encouraging verbalization of fears, teaching principles related to nutrition, and providing a bed bath also are examples of specific independent nursing interventions. *Interdependent interventions* are actions implemented in collaboration with other appropriate professionals. An example of an interdependent intervention is implementing actions identified in standing orders or a protocol. These situations delineate the parameters within which the nurse is permitted to administer to the patient. Protocols and standing orders are commonly found in emergency and critical care areas.

SAMPLE ITEM 4–27

The charge nurse assigns the staff nurse to insert a Foley catheter. The first action by the nurse is to:

(1) Explain the procedure to the patient

(2) Gather all equipment at the bedside

(3) Check the physician's order

(4) Wash hands thoroughly

This question is designed to test your ability to recognize that the insertion of a Foley catheter is a dependent nursing intervention that requires a physician's order. Knowing what actions are dependent, independent, and interdependent are types of nursing actions that can be tested.

Methods of Implementation

Nursing care is delivered by using various implementation methods such as assisting with ADLs; counseling and teaching; implementing strategies to achieve outcomes such as responding to adverse reactions, implementing preventive measures, preparing a patient for a procedure, performing a procedure and implementing lifesaving actions; supervising and evaluating the effectiveness of delegated interventions; and sharing results of nursing actions verbally and in writing.

Providing for or assisting with ADLs refers to activities associated with eating, dressing, hygiene, grooming, toileting, transfer, and locomotion. Situations associated with needs addressing ADLs can be acute, chronic, temporary, permanent, or related to maintaining or restoring function. The activities of daily living are an integral part of life and therefore are emphasized.

Teaching and counseling enables the nurse to assist a patient to accept actual or evolving changes that are caused by loss, illness, disability, or stress. To effectively teach in the cognitive (learning new information), psychomotor (learning new skills), and affective (developing new attitudes, values, and beliefs) domains, the nurse must apply teaching-learning principles to motivate patients to learn and grow. To effectively counsel, the nurse must apply therapeutic communication principles to explore feelings and meet patients' emotional needs. People are complex human beings and care must comprehensively address the physical, emotional and mental realms.

To assist patients to achieve therapeutic goals, the nurse must implement preventive measures and identify and respond to adverse reactions or life-threatening situations. Preventive actions are those activities that help the patient avoid a health problem. Administering immunizations, indicating on the identification bracelet that the patient is allergic to a specific drug, and providing health teaching are examples of preventive measures. An example of identifying and responding to adverse reactions would be stopping the administration of an antibiotic in response to a patient's allergic reaction. Initiating cardiopulmonary resuscitation, implementing the abdominal thrust (Heimlich maneuver), or administering emergency medications are examples of measures that can be implemented in life-threatening situations. Most of these interventions address basic physiological needs required for survival and are therefore frequently tested.

Preparing patients physically and emotionally for a diagnostic test, procedure, or surgery or correctly implementing a procedure are components of implementing nursing care. The nurse must know how and when to implement a procedure and the expected outcomes of the procedure. Inserting a Foley catheter, providing a tube feeding, and administering an enema are examples of procedures implemented by the nurse. Because nursing care often involves *laying on of the hands,* procedures and psychomotor skills are frequently tested.

Providing an environment that supports the achievement of health care goals and/or outcomes is also an important component of implementation. Providing for privacy, promoting a motivating climate, accepting feelings, and providing for environmental safety all contribute to a supportive environment. Supportive environments influence both the physical and emotional status of patients. Concepts related to maintaining a therapeutic environment are commonly tested principles because they are second-level needs identified by Maslow.

Occasionally the nurse who formulates the plan of care delegates all or part of the implementation of that care to other members of the nursing team. Uncomplicated and basic interventions, particularly those associated with activities of daily living, are often delegated to a nurse aide or licensed practical nurse. The nurse who delegates is responsible for the plan of care and is accountable for ensuring that the plan of care is delivered according to standards of the profession.

SAMPLE ITEM 4–28

The patient has an order for a low-sodium diet. Of the following items on the meal tray, the nurse teaches the patient to avoid:

(1) Salt

(2) Sugar

(3) Liquids

(4) Margarine

This item tests your ability to identify a principle that needs to be taught to a patient. Teaching is an implementation method used by the nurse to assist a patient to meet an identified expected outcome. Mainly, this question tests your ability to recognize that salt is sodium, and therefore, should be avoided by a patient on a low-sodium diet.

SAMPLE ITEM 4–29

When a patient vomits while in the supine position, the nurse should:

(1) Raise the patient to a high-Fowler's position

(2) Transfer the patient to the bathroom

(3) Position the head between the knees

(4) Turn the patient on the side.

This item is designed to test your ability to appropriately respond to an event. To answer this question, you need to recognize that it is important to quickly assist the patient to expectorate the vomitus to avoid aspiration. In addition, you need to know that turning the patient on the side is the best position to facilitate drainage of matter from the mouth. Responding to an event by implementing an action is an implementation question.

SAMPLE ITEM 4–30

To provide support for the patient who complains of nausea, the nurse should:

(1) Give mouth care every shift

(2) Delay meals until the nausea passes

(3) Position the emesis basin in easy reach

(4) Explain that the nausea will lessen with time

Implementing actions that anticipate an event is the step of implementation, not planning. The word "provide" in the stem gives you a clue that this is an implementation question. To answer this question correctly, you need to know that a complaint of nausea is a precursor to vomiting and that providing an emesis basin will provide physical and emotional support to the nauseated patient.

SAMPLE ITEM 4–31

The underlying rationale for turning a patient every 2 hours is to:

(1) Relieve pressure

(2) Assess skin condition

(3) Ensure that skin is clean and dry

(4) Provide massage to bony prominences

This item tests your ability to recognize the correct rationale for a nursing procedure. To implement safe and effective care, nurses need to have a strong understanding of the scientific rationales for nursing actions.

SAMPLE ITEM 4–32

When administering medications, the safest way to identify a patient is to:

(1) Ask the patient his or her name

(2) Look at the name on the bed

(3) Check the identification bracelet

(4) Call the patient's name and observe the response

This test item is designed to see if you can correctly identify a step in a procedure. While more than one of the options might be an action implemented by the nurse, the question is asking you to choose the best answer from all the options offered. In this set of options, checking the identification bracelet is the most reliable and safest method to verify a patient's identity.

SAMPLE ITEM 4–33

To provide aseptically safe perineal care to a female patient, the nurse should:

(1) Use different parts of the cloth with each stroke

(2) Apply deodorant spray to the perineal area

(3) Cleanse the labia in a circular motion

(4) Sprinkle talcum powder on the perineum

This item tests your ability to identify a correct step in a procedure. To answer this question correctly, you also need to know what actions related to perineal care are based on a microbiological principal. Identifying a step in a procedure is a question designed to test your knowledge of implementing a nursing measure based on a scientific principle.

SAMPLE ITEM 4–34

The charge nurse delegates the implementation of a nasogastric tube feeding to a licensed practical nurse (LPN). Which of the following statements is accurate in terms of the responsibility of the charge nurse?

(1) The charge should implement the planned care and not delegate

(2) The LPN should respectfully refuse to implement this care

(3) The charge nurse is responsible for delegated care

(4) The LPN is accountable for one's own actions

This item tests your ability to recognize that a nurse who delegates care to another staff member is responsible for supervising and evaluating the delivery of that care. This is an important component of implementation and is a concept that is often tested.

Documenting and Reporting Patient Care and Responses

Once care is delivered, it is recorded along with an assessment of the patient's response to care. In addition to documenting care given, the nurse may verbally share results with other health team members. Verbal reports are usually given when changing shifts; responding to an emergency; and reporting abnormal responses to care.

SAMPLE ITEM 4–35

When the nurse signs a turning and positioning schedule form, it indicates that the patient:

(1) Received a back rub with lotion

(2) Was turned at the time initialed

(3) Received passive range-of-motion exercises

(4) Was encouraged to turn to a different position

     This question tests your ability to recognize the purpose of a turning and positioning flow sheet. Documenting care given is a component of the step of implementation.

EVALUATION

Evaluation is the fifth and final step of the nursing process. Evaluation is a process that consists of four steps that must be implemented after care plan is delivered if effectiveness of the nursing care plan is to be determined. The evaluation process includes identifying patient responses to care; comparing a patient's actual responses to the expected outcomes; analyzing factors that affected the actual outcomes for the purpose of drawing conclusions about the success or failure of specific nursing activities; and modifying the nursing care plan when necessary. Evaluation items will ask you to:

- Identify the steps in the evaluation process
- Identify actual outcomes as being desirable or undesirable
- Identify whether an outcome in a situation is met or not met
- Identify progress or lack of progress toward an expected outcome
- Recognize the need to modify the nursing care plan in response to a change in the status of the patient or a plan that is ineffective
- Recognize that the process of evaluation is continuous
- Recognize that the nursing process is dynamic and cyclical

Critical words used within a test item that generally indicate that the item is focused on evaluation include "expected," "met," "desired," "compared," "succeeded," "failed," "achieved," "modified," "reassess," "ineffective," "effective," "response," "compliance," "noncompliance," and "evaluate." See if you can identify variations of these critical words indicating evaluation activities in the sample items. Most testing errors occur during the evaluation phase of the nursing process when options are selected that:

- Do not thoroughly and accurately reassess the patient after care is implemented
- Fail to appropriately cluster new data
- Fail to determine significance of new data
- Come to inappropriate or inaccurate conclusions
- Fail to modify the nursing care plan in response to the changing needs of the patient or in response to an ineffective plan

Identifying Patient Responses

The process of evaluation begins with a reassessment that collects new information. Once nursing care is implemented, the patient is reassessed and new clusters of data are identified and significance determined. In the nursing literature, the term "evaluation" has often been used interchangeably with the term "assessment," which causes confusion. It is important to remember that assessment is only one component in the process of evaluation. The nurse needs to first reassess to identify patient outcomes. Patient outcomes are the actual patient responses to nursing care. These data are then clustered and their significance determined before these actual patient outcomes can be compared with expected outcomes.

SAMPLE ITEM 4–36

A patient on a bland diet complains that she has a poor appetite. The MOST effective way to assess if the patient's nutritional needs have been met would be to:

(1) Institute a 3-day food intake study
(2) Weigh the patient at the end of the week
(3) Request an order for a dietary assessment
(4) Compare a current weight with the weight history

This item is designed to test your ability to identify a common way to evaluate a patient's nutritional status. In this situation the results of nutritional care are determined by comparing a current weight assessment with a previous weight assessment in an effort to identify any gain or loss in the patient's weight. Once a change in status is identified, a conclusion about the effectiveness of care can be determined from the data.

Comparing Actual Outcomes with Expected Outcomes

Patient outcomes are the criteria that are established for evaluation of nursing care. A comparison is made between the actual outcomes and the expected outcomes to determine the effectiveness of nursing intervention. The new data when compared with expected outcomes determine which outcomes have been achieved and those that have not been achieved. The closer the patient's actual outcomes are to expected outcomes, the more positive the evaluation. Negative evaluations are based on the fact that actual outcomes did not achieve expected outcomes. Negative evaluations indicate that an error occurred in the implementation of the nursing process or nursing care was ineffective. An example of a positive evaluation would be when the nurse crushes and mixes medication with applesauce expecting that the patient will have less difficulty swallowing the medication. Following administration, the nurse determines that this intervention was effective because the patient had no difficulty swallowing the medication.

SAMPLE ITEM 4–37

The nurse would know that the patient understood the teaching about a low-sodium diet when from a menu the patient selects:

(1) Milk

(2) Fruit

(3) Celery

(4) Vegetables

This item is designed to test your ability to recognize that of all the options presented, fruit has the least amount of sodium. In addition, the stem is worded in such a way that it requires the nurse to evaluate the correctness of the patient's response. The action described in the stem is an attempt to evaluate the patient's understanding of the teaching provided.

Analyzing Factors That Affect Actual Outcomes of Care

Once a determination of whether care is effective or not is made, then the nurse must come to some conclusions about the potential factors that contributed to the success or failure of the nursing care plan. If a plan of care is ineffective, the nurse must examine what contributed to its failure. This requires the nurse to start at step 1 of the nursing process with assessment and work through the entire process again in an attempt to identify why the plan was ineffective. Questions the nurse must ask include "Was the original assessment accurate?" "Was the nursing diagnosis accurate, and did it include all the *related-to*-factors?" "Was the goal realistic?" "Were the outcomes measurable?" "Were the interventions consistently implemented?" When plans of care fail because *related-to* factors used in the NANDA terminology were incorrectly identified or omitted, then nursing strategies generally were inappropriate or were never implemented.

to page 73

SAMPLE ITEM 4-38

A patient returns to the clinic after taking a 7-day course of antibiotic therapy and is still exhibiting signs of an urinary tract infection. The nurse's initial action should be to:

(1) Obtain another urine specimen for a culture and sensitivity

(2) Determine if the patient took the medication as prescribed

(3) Arrange for the physician to order a different antibiotic

(4) Make an appointment for the patient to be seen by the physician

This item is designed to test your ability to recognize that the nurse must analyze the factors that influence outcomes of care. Options 3 and 4 can be eliminated because these actions immediately move to an intervention before collecting more information. Option 1 can be deleted because it may be unnecessary depending on the information gleaned from option 2. Option 2 is the correct answer because compliance with a medication administration schedule will influence the effectiveness of the medication.

Modifying the Nursing Care Plan

Once it is determined that a plan of care is ineffective, the plan must be modified. The changes in the plan of care are based on new patient assessments, nursing diagnoses, goals, and/or nursing strategies that are designed to address the specific needs of the patient. The modified plan must then be implemented, and the whole evaluation process begins again. As one can see, the process of evaluation is continuous.

to page 74

```
╔══════════════════════════════════════════╗
║ ▓▓▓ SAMPLE ITEM 4–39 ▓▓▓                   ║
╚══════════════════════════════════════════╝
```

SAMPLE ITEM 4–39

A newly admitted patient was provided with a regular diet consisting of three traditional meals a day. After a week it was identified that the patient was only eating approximately 50 percent of her meals and was losing weight. The nurse should:

(1) Schedule several between-meal supplements

(2) Assist the patient until meals are completed

(3) Change the care plan to provide five small meals daily

(4) Secure an order to increase the number of calories provided

This item is designed to test your ability to recognize that the nursing care plan must be changed when care is ineffective. Option 1 is eliminated because it is a dependent intervention and requires a physician's order. Option 4 is eliminated because the patient presently has difficulty completing what is on the tray. Option 2 is eliminated because the nurse does not have a right to force the patient to eat everything on the meal tray. Option 3 identifies an independent function of the nurse that does not require a physician's order. Small frequent feedings spread the meals throughout the day and provide a smaller volume at each meal. Psychologically this is not as overwhelming as attempting to consume a full meal. Small frequent meals are motivating because consuming the smaller volume is more realistic and achievable. Ineffective nursing care must be modified until patient needs are met.

ANSWERS AND RATIONALES FOR SAMPLE ITEMS IN CHAPTER 4

An asterisk (*) is in front of the rationale that explains the correct answer.

Assessment

4–1 * (1) An assessment must be made to determine if any intervention is necessary to stabilize an injured body part prior to moving a patient; moving an injured person could exacerbate an injury.

(2) Moving an injured patient before assessment and stabilization could exacerbate an injury.

(3) Same as #2.

(4) This would be done after the patient is safe; this does not address the need for an immediate assessment of the patient's condition.

4–2 * (1) Nurses must always assess a patient prior to activity to ensure that the patient has the strength to safely ambulate.

(2) This is concerned with implementing care; the patient's strength must be assessed before ambulating to determine if it is safe.

(3) Same as #2.

(4) The patient's strength must be assessed before the transfer to the wheelchair; not all patients using a wheelchair need a vest restraint to maintain safety.

4–3 (1) These are within the normal range.

(2) Same as #1.

(3) Same as #1.

* (4) These are outside the normal range; normal respirations are 14 to 20, effortless, and noiseless; this patient may be having respiratory distress.

4–4 (1) A nurse may permit an alert and capable patient to insert a rectal thermometer; however, if the patient has physical or cognitive deficits, this may not be possible.

(2) When taking a rectal temperature, the patient can be safely positioned on either the right or left side.

(3) The use of an electronic thermometer is not always practical; electronic thermometers are usually not used in isolation because of the inconvenience related to the need to decontaminate equipment after use.

* (4) This is always done to facilitate thermometer entry; a lubricant reduces resistance when inserting a thermometer past the anal sphincter.

4–5 * (1) To calculate ideal body weight, the nurse needs to know the patient's height, age, and extent of bone structure.

(2) This reflects the amount of food the patient is ingesting; this information does not contribute to the calculation of ideal body weight.

(3) This is determined by weight and inches reflecting circumference of the chest and waist; this information does not contribute to the calculation of ideal body weight.

(4) This supports the patient's right to make choices about care; this information does not contribute to the calculation of ideal body weight.

4–6 (1) Data are classified as objective or subjective, not primary. "Primary" refers to a source of data; a patient is the primary source of data.

(2 These data can be measured or assessed by one of the senses.

(3) Types of data are classified as objective or subjective, not secondary. "Secondary" refers to sources of data; a secondary source of data produces information from a source other than the patient.

* (4) Subjective data are collected when the patient shares feelings, perceptions, sensations, and thoughts.

4–7 (1) The wife is a secondary source, not a primary source.

(2) The wife is a secondary source, not a tertiary source.

* (3) Family members are secondary sources. Secondary sources produce information from someplace other than the patient. Secondary sources provide supplemental information about the patient.

(4) The wife is not a subjective source. "Subjective" refers to a type of data; subjective data are collected when the patient shares feelings, perceptions, sensations, and thoughts about a health problem.

4–8 (1) This is considered verbal; words are written.

* (2) This is nonverbal. A message is transmitted without using words; crying, facial expressions, and the patient's appearance are further examples of nonverbal communication.

(3) Sounds may or may not communicate meaning; a sound which communicates a meaning is considered verbal communication.

(4) This is verbal communication; words are generally spoken in a telephone message.

4–9 (1) This would indicate concentrated urine; reduced fluid intake will cause urine to be dark straw colored.

* (2) This is the normal color of urine; this color indicates that a patient is receiving adequate fluid intake.

(3) This may reflect concentrated urine, an infection, or a small amount of blood in the urine.

(4) This may reflect very concentrated urine, an infection, or blood in the urine.

4–10 (1) This is done once the initial blood pressure is verified; once one vital sign is identified as abnormal, all the vital signs should be assessed.

* (2) The reading should be verified by retaking the blood pressure because the nurse may have made a mistake when originally taking the blood pressure.

(3) This may be done after the blood pressure is verified and all the vital signs are taken.

(4) Same as #3.

4–11 (1) Vital signs dramatically outside normal parameters, such as asystole or apnea, would trigger a code, not vital signs just outside normal parameters.

* (2) The physician needs to be notified of significant patient adaptations to respond with a medical plan.

(3) The supervisor is not legally permitted to respond with medical orders; only a licensed physician can order interventions such as medications to alter a blood pressure; although the supervisor may be informed of the status of the patient, it is not the best option offered in this test item.

(4) This is unsafe; unexpected abnormal vital signs require more frequent assessment and immediate medical action.

Analysis

4–12 (1) This is related to an inability to communicate basic thoughts either in writing or verbally; it is not related to a potential for aspiration.

* (2) This could contribute to a potential for aspiration; it is related to the data identified in the stem and together presents a cluster of information that is significant.

(3) This is not related to the data cluster identified in the stem; this is related to the inability of the patient to provide for self-care.

(4) This is not related to the data cluster identified in the stem; this is related to hygiene needs and supports the fact that the patient is at risk for altered skin integrity, not aspiration.

4–13 * (1) Patients who are immobilized are subject to increased pressure over bony prominences with subsequent decrease in circulation to tissues.

(2) This is unrelated to the development of decubitus ulcers.

(3) Same as #2.

(4) Same as #2.

4–14 (1) Acting-out behaviors are most commonly reflective of anger.
  (2) Refusing to believe or accept a situation, not depressive behaviors, are reflective of denial.
* (3) Depression is commonly exhibited by patients in such behaviors as avoiding contact with others, withdrawing, not eating (anorexia), and not sleeping (insomnia).
  (4) Acceptance is related to the final step of grieving; a patient reconciles and accepts the situation and is at peace within the self.

4–15 (1) The patient is seeking independence, not trying to be left alone.
  (2) The primary motivation for this behavior is to feel independent, not to belong or be accepted.
* (3) This is correct; the patient is attempting to perform self-care to demonstrate the ability to be self-sufficient.
  (4) The patient is seeking independence, not trying to manipulate the staff.

4–16 * (1) These patient adaptations are related to a decreased blood volume associated with postoperative hemorrhage.
  (2) With this process the patient would more likely be hypertensive with a rapid pulse.
  (3) Same as #2.
  (4) Same as #2.

4–17 (1) This is a need, not a nursing diagnosis.
  (2) This is a combination of an expected outcome and an intervention, not a nursing diagnosis.
  (3) This is an incorrectly worded nursing diagnosis; a stroke is not something a nurse can treat.
* (4) This is an appropriately worded nursing diagnosis that uses NANDA terminology; it contains a health problem appropriate for nursing interventions.

4–18 * (1) The nurse has an obligation to ensure that all patients' needs will be appropriately met; this is the only option that addresses this concept.
  (2) This is inappropriate; all patients must have their needs met.
  (3) This is inappropriate; once the nurse assumes a course of duty, the nurse is responsible for the care that is delivered.
  (4) This action does not ensure that appropriate care will be provided; this action will increase anxiety and cause patients to doubt the quality of care being provided.

Planning

4–19 (1) This is a long-term goal, not a short-term goal.
  (2) This is correct wording for a goal, but it is unrealistic; goals should be patient centered, specific, measurable, have a time frame, and be realistic.
* (3) This is a short-term goal; it is patient centered, specific, and measurable; "remain" reflects the time frame.
  (4) This is the problem statement, not a goal.

4–20 * (1) Providing for a patient's oxygenation is essential to maintain life and is always the priority.
  (2) This is important; however, providing for a patent airway takes priority.

(3) Same as #2.

(4) Same as #2.

4–21 * (1) Measures such as covering a cough, frequent handwashing, and correct disposal of soiled tissues can limit the spread of microorganisms.

(2) This is unnecessary; it is used only when a patient has an extremely virulent microorganism.

(3) Antibiotics are usually not given to prevent infection, but to treat an infection.

(4) This is unnecessary; fresh air does not spread the flu.

4–22 * (1) An occupied bed is made for a patient on complete bed rest; this patient is not permitted out of bed.

(2) This is unnecessary; an occupied bed can be made with minimal strain to the patient.

(3) This is inappropriate; all the linens should be changed regularly and whenever necessary.

(4) This is unsafe; a patient on bed rest is not allowed out of bed for any reason unless otherwise directed by a physician's order.

4–23 (1) This patient can be transferred out of bed while the linen is changed.

(2) Same as #1.

(3) Same as #1.

* (4) Patients on bed rest must remain in bed when the linens are changed; this is called "making an occupied bed."

4–24 * (1) This is a correctly stated expected outcome; it is patient centered, measurable, and has a stated date of completion.

(2) This is the problem statement of a nursing diagnosis, not an expected outcome.

(3) This is the nurse's goal, not an expected outcome.

(4) This is a planned intervention, not an expected outcome.

4–25 (1) This will increase the demand on the patient's respiratory system. This increases activity which in turn increases oxygen needs; rushing may cause the patient to become upset.

(2) This does not address the patient's respiratory needs; a full bath may be needed by the patient.

* (3) This action conserves energy; rest periods reduce the strain of activity by decreasing the demand for oxygenation, which in turn decreases the rate and labor of respirations.

(4) The patient's dyspnea cannot be ignored; the plan must be changed to allow for rest periods to reduce the physical demand for oxygen.

4–26 (1) When a patient is unresponsive to common nursing interventions, the nurse needs to consult with an expert nurse, not a medical specialist.

(2) The physical therapist is a specialist in the area of assisting a patient to achieve or maintain physical mobility; the nurse needs to consult with an expert nurse, not a physical therapist.

(3) The physician is responsible for the patient's medical care and is not an expert in providing nursing care.

* (4) The clinical nurse specialist is educated and prepared to provide expert assistance when other members of the health team seek solutions to difficult clinical nursing problems.

Implementation

4–27 (1) This occurs once the order is verified.

(2) This occurs after the order is verified and the procedure is explained to the patient.

* (3) This is a dependent nursing intervention and requires a physician's order that must be verified by the nurse implementing the order.

(4) This is done once the order is verified and explained to the patient.

4–28* (1) Salt used to season meals contains sodium; sodium must be avoided when a patient is on a low-sodium diet.

(2) Sugar is avoided when a patient is on a reduced-calorie or diabetic diet, not when on a low-sodium diet.

(3) Fluids need to be avoided when the patient is on fluid restriction, not when on a low-sodium diet; however, the patient must be alert to avoid fluids that are high in sodium such as diet sodas.

(4) Margarine is avoided when a patient is on a low-fat diet, not when on a low-sodium diet.

4–29 (1) This position does not facilitate the exit of vomitus from the mouth.

(2) This is unsafe; vomiting takes energy and could cause the patient to become weak during transfer.

(3) This does not support or protect the vomiting patient; this position is often used to increase cerebral perfusion when a person feels dizzy, not to facilitate vomiting.

* (4) This drains the mouth via gravity and reduces the risk of aspiration.

4–30 (1) This is unnecessary; daily mouth care is sufficient unless the patient is vomiting and then more frequent mouth care is indicated.

(2) This is inappropriate; nausea may be a long-standing problem.

* (3) This provides for physical and emotional comfort; the emesis basin collects vomitus rather than soiling the bed linens and reduces the patient's concern regarding soiling.

(4) This is false reassurance; the nurse cannot predict when nausea will subside.

4–31 * (1) Turning relieves pressure from body weight and permits circulation to return to the area; prolonged pressure can cause cell death from lack of oxygen and nutrients needed to sustain cellular metabolism.

(2) While this should be done, relieving pressure is the main purpose of regularly turning and positioning a patient.

(3) Same as #2.

(4) Same as #2.

4–32 (1) This is unsafe; the patient could be cognitively impaired.

(2) This is unsafe; the patient could be in the wrong bed.

* (3) This is the safest method to identify a patient; it is the most reliable because each patient on admission receives an identification bracelet with his or her name and an identification number.

(4) Same as #1.

4–33 * (1) This provides a clean surface for each stroke when washing; this avoids contaminating the meatus with soiled portions of the cloth.

(2) This can be irritating, contribute to the risk of impaired skin integrity, and does not remove bacteria.

(3) This is unsafe; this would bring soiled matter into contact with the urinary meatus; washing from the pubis to the rectum using a clean portion of the cloth with each stroke, not circular motions, limits contamination of the meatus.

(4) Same as #2.

4–34 (1) This is unnecessary; a nurse can delegate tasks to other nursing staff members as long as delegated tasks are supervised and their delivery evaluated.

(2) It is inappropriate to refuse to implement delegated tasks as long as the tasks are within the legal definition of LPN practice and the LPN can safely implement the task; the question is asking which of the options is accurate in terms of the responsibiity of the charge nurse, not the LPN.

* (3) This is an accurate statement; the delegating nurse is responsible for supervising and evaluating the delivery of delegated tasks.

(4) This is a true statement; however, the question is asking which of the options is accurate in terms of the responsibility of the charge nurse, not the LPN.

4–35 (1) While a backrub should be implemented when a patient is turned and positioned, the turning and positioning sheet only indicates that the patient was turned and positioned.

* (2) This indicates that turning and positioning were implemented as planned.

(3) A turning and positioning flow sheet documents turning and positioning, not passive range-of-motion exercises.

(4) A patient must actually be turned and positioned before the nurse signs the turning and positioning flow sheet; while a patient might be encouraged to turn, it does not mean that the patient was actually turned.

Evaluation

4–36 (1) This might be done after it is determined that the patient has lost weight.

(2) It is unnecessary to wait a full week; the patient's nutritional status immediately can be assessed by comparing a current weight with the patient's weight history.

(3) Same as #1.

* (4) Measuring a patient's weight and comparing the weight with a previous weight is an easy and quick way to assess a patient's nutritional status.

4–37   (1) This has more sodium than fruit.
     * (2) Fruit has the least amount of sodium compared to the distractors.
        (3) Same as #1.
        (4) Same as #1.

4–38   (1) This would be inappropriate before collecting additional data related to the present plan of care; this may be necessary later.
     * (2) Determining compliance with the medical regimen is the priority; antibiotics must be taken routinely and consistently to maintain adequate blood levels of the drug.
        (3) Same as #1.
        (4) Same as #1.

4–39   (1) This action is a dependent function and requires a physician's order.
        (2) Patients must not be forced to eat all their meals; the portions may be too large for the anorexic patient to ingest.
     * (3) This action is an independent function of the nurse and does not require a physician's order; small frequent feedings spread the meals throughout the day and provide a volume that is not as overwhelming as a full meal.
        (4) The problem is not the number of calories provided on the tray but the amount of food the patient is able to ingest at any one time. Small frequent feedings spread the meals throughout the day and provide a volume that is not as overwhelming as a full meal.

5 Test-Taking Techniques

Performing well on multiple-choice questions requires both roots and wings. The previous chapters were concerned with factors that provided you with roots. Each root grounded you through information about formulating a positive mental attitude, exploring a variety of study skills, introducing you to the multiple-choice question, and familiarizing you with the nursing process. This chapter attempts to provide you with the wings necessary to accurately fly through multiple-choice questions. Flying through multiple-choice questions has nothing to do with speed; it relates to being test-wise and able to navigate through complex information with ease.

Tests in nursing involve complex information that has depth and breadth. As well as having its own body of knowledge, nursing draws from a variety of disciplines, such as sociology, psychology, and anatomy and physiology. To perform well on a nursing examination, you must understand and integrate the subject matter. Nothing can replace effective study habits or knowledge about the subject being tested. However, being testwise can maximize the application of the information you possess.

Being test-wise entails specific techniques related to individual question analysis and general techniques related to conquering the challenge of an examination. One rationale for learning how to utilize these techniques is to provide you with skills that increase your command over the testing situation. If you are in control, you will maintain a positive attitude and increase your chances of selecting the correct answers. When you have knowledge and are test-wise, you should fly through a test by gliding and soaring, rather than by flapping and fluttering.

SPECIFIC TEST-TAKING TECHNIQUES

A specific test-taking technique is a strategy that uses skill and forethought to analyze a test item before selecting an answer. A technique is not a gimmick but a method of examining a question with consideration and thoughtfulness. Hopefully, the outcome will be the selection of the correct answer. When an item has four options, the chance of selecting the correct answer is one out of four, or 25 percent. When you eliminate one distractor, the chance of selecting the correct answer is one out of three, or 33.3 percent. If you are able to throw out two distractors, the chance of selecting the correct answer is one out of two, or 50 percent. Each time you successfully eliminate a distractor, you dramatically increase your chances of correctly answering the question.

Before you attempt to answer a question, break the question down into its components. First, read the stem. What is it actually asking? It may be helpful to paraphrase the stem to focus in on its content. Then, try to answer the question being asked in your own words before looking at the options. Hopefully, one of the options will be similar to your answer. Then examine the other options and try to identify the correct answer. If you know, understand, and can apply the information being tested, you can often recognize the correct answer. However, do not be tempted to rapidly select an option without careful thought. An option may contain accurate information, but it may not be correct because it does not answer the question asked in the stem. Be careful. Each option deserves equal consideration.

Use test-taking techniques for every question. The use of test-taking techniques becomes paramount when you are unsure of the answer because each distractor that you are able to eliminate will increase your chances of selecting the correct answer. Most nursing students are able to reduce the number of plausible answers to two. However, contrary to popular belief, multiple-choice questions in nursing have only one correct answer. Use everything in your arsenal to conquer the multiple-choice question test: effective studying; a positive mental attitude; and last but not least test-taking techniques.

For your information the correct answers for the sample items in this chapter and the rationales for all the options are at the end of this chapter.

Identify Key Words in the Stem That Indicate Negative Polarity

Read the stem slowly and precisely. Look for key words such as "not," "except," "never," "contraindicated," "unacceptable," "avoid," and "least." These words indicate negative polarity, and the question being asked is probably concerned with what is false. Some words that have negative polarity are not as obvious as others. A negatively worded stem asks you to identify an exception, detect an error, or recognize nursing interventions that are unacceptable or contraindicated. If you read a stem and all the options appear correct, reread the stem because you may have missed a key negative word. These words are sometimes brought to your attention by an underline (<u>not</u>), italics (*except*), boldface (**never**), or capitals (VIOLATE). Many nursing examinations avoid questions with negative polarity. However, examples of these items are included for your information.

to page 85

SAMPLE ITEM 5–1

Which of the following would violate medical asepsis when making an occupied bed?

(1) Wearing gloves when changing the linen

(2) Returning unused linen to the linen closet

(3) Using the old top sheet for the new bottom sheet

(4) Tucking clean linen against the springs of the bed

The key term in this stem is *violate*. The stem is asking you to identify the option that does not follow correct medical aseptic technique. If you misread the stem and were looking for the answer that indicated correct medical aseptic technique, then there would be more than one correct answer. When this happens, reread the stem for a word with negative polarity. In this item you had to be particularly careful because the word "violate" is not emphasized for your attention.

SAMPLE ITEM 5–2

A patient is on a low-sodium diet. Prior to discharge he or she should be taught to *avoid*:

(1) Stewed fruit

(2) Luncheon meats

(3) Whole-grain cereal

(4) Green leafy vegetables

The key word in this stem is *avoid*. The stem is asking you to select the food that a patient on a low-sodium diet should not eat. If you misread the question and were looking for foods that are permitted on a low-sodium diet, then there would be more than one correct answer. When there appears to be more than one answer, reread the stem for a key negative word that you may have missed.

SAMPLE ITEM 5–3

When rubbing a patient's back, the nurse should NEVER:
(1) Knead the skin
(2) Wipe off excess lotion
(3) Use a continuous firm stroke
(4) Put pressure over the vertebrae

The key word in this stem is *never.* The stem is asking you to identify which option is not an acceptable practice associated with a backrub. If you missed the word NEVER and were looking for what the nurse should do for a backrub, then there would be more than one correct answer. This should clue you to the fact that you may have missed a key negative word.

Identify Key Words in the Stem That Set a Priority

Read the stem carefully while looking for key words such as "first," "initially," "best," and "most." These words modify what is being asked. This type of question requires you to put a value on each option and then place them in rank order. If the question asks what should the nurse do first, the initial action by the nurse should be, or the best response would be, then rank the options in order of importance from 1 to 4 with the most desirable option as number 1 and the least desirable option as number 4. The correct answer would be the option that you ranked number 1. If you are having difficulty ranking the options, eliminate the option that you believe is most wrong among all the options. Next, eliminate the option you believe is most wrong from among the remaining three options. At this point you are down to two options and your chance of selecting the correct answer is 50 percent. When key words such as "most important" are used, frequently all of the options may be appropriate nursing care for the situation; however, only one of the options is the most important. When all the options appear logical for the situation, reread the stem to identify a key word that asks you to place a priority on the options. These words are occasionally emphasized by an underline, *italics,* **boldface,** or CAPITALS.

to page 87

SAMPLE ITEM 5–4

The nurse is assigned to care for a patient who is incontinent of urine and stool. To *best* protect the skin, the nurse should apply:

(1) A petroleum-type jelly

(2) An incontinence pad

(3) Talcum powder

(4) Corn starch

The key term in this stem is *best.* Each of these options is something a nurse might do for the incontinent patient. The stem is asking you to place a value on each option and decide which nursing intervention best protects the skin when compared to the other options. If you are having difficulty ranking these options, eliminate the option that is most wrong. Although an incontinence pad absorbs urine and is often used for incontinent patients, it holds excreta next to the skin and actually promotes skin breakdown. Eliminate option 2. Continue to eliminate options you believe are wrong, and then make your final selection for the correct answer.

SAMPLE ITEM 5–5

Prior to administering an enema, the nurse's <u>first</u> action should be to:

(1) Verify the physician's order

(2) Collect the appropriate equipment

(3) Arrange for the bathroom to be empty

(4) Inform the patient about the procedure

The key word in this stem is *first.* Each of these options includes a step that is part of the procedure for administering an enema. You must decide which option is the first step among the four options presented. Before you can teach a patient, collect equipment, or actually administer the enema, you need to know the type of enema ordered. The type of enema will influence the other steps of the procedure. If option 1 were different, such as use medical asepsis to dispose of contaminated articles, then the correct answer among these four options would be option 4. You can only choose the first step of a procedure from among the options presented.

SAMPLE ITEM 5–6

The nurse observes another nurse treating a patient in an abusive manner. The nurse's *initial* action should be to:

(1) Tell the charge nurse and write a report
(2) Become a role model for the other nurse
(3) Talk with the nurse about the incident
(4) Reassure and calm the patient

The key word in this stem is *initial.* All the options in this question are appropriate nursing interventions for this situation. The stem is asking you to identify what the nurse should do initially or first. The correct answer may not be the best intervention for dealing with the abusive nurse, but that is not what the question is asking. It is asking what should be the nurse's initial action in this situation. The question is testing your ability to recognize that the patient's physical and emotional safety is the priority.

SAMPLE ITEM 5–7

Mr. Vost has significant short-term memory loss and does not remember his primary nurse from day to day. When the patient asks, "Who are you?" the most appropriate response would be:

(1) "You know me. I take care of you every day."
(2) To say nothing, because it would only get him upset.
(3) "Don't worry. I'm the same nurse you had yesterday."
(4) "My name is Sue Clark. I am the nurse caring for you."

The key words in this stem are *most appropriate.* Potential responses are reflected in this question. You are asked to select the best or most suitable response from among the four options presented. You may dislike all of the statements. You may even think of a response that you personally prefer to the offered options. You cannot rewrite the question. You must select your answer from the options presented in the item. The words "most appropriate" are not highlighted in this item, and therefore you must be diligent when reading the stem.

Identify Clues in the Stem

A clue is the unintentional use of a word or phrase that leads you to the correct answer. Generally the stem is short and contains only the information needed to make it clear and specific. Therefore, a word or phrase in the stem may provide a hint for choosing the correct answer. A word that is a clue in the stem may be identical or similar to a word used in the correct answer. When a word is identical in the stem and the answer, it is called a *clang association.* A phrase that is a clue in the stem is usually paraphrased in or closely related to the correct answer.

SAMPLE ITEM 5–8

Psychosocial development is most influenced by:
(1) Food
(2) Alcohol
(3) Society
(4) Genetics

An important word in the stem is *psychosocial.* When examining the options, one of them contains the word "society." Society is closely related to psychosocial. Carefully consider this option. More often than not it will be the correct answer.

SAMPLE ITEM 5–9

To help meet a patient's self-esteem needs, the nurse should:
(1) Encourage the patient to perform self-care when able
(2) Suggest that the family visit the patient more often
(3) Anticipate needs before the patient requests help
(4) Assist the patient with bathing and grooming

An important word in the stem is *self-esteem.* The word "self-esteem" is similar to the word "self-care." Thoughtfully examine option 1. An option that incorporates words that are similar to words in the stem is often the correct answer.

to page 90

SAMPLE ITEM 5–10

To meet a patient's basic physical needs, the nurse should:
(1) Pull the curtain when providing care
(2) Answer the call bell immediately
(3) Administer physical hygiene
(4) Obtain vital signs

An important word in the stem is *physical.* It is an unintentional clue that should provide a hint that option 3 is the correct answer. The use of the word "physical" in both the stem and the option is called a *clang association.* It is the repetitious use of a word. Examine option 3 because when a clang association occurs, it is often the correct answer.

Identify Patient-Centered Options

Nursing is a profession that is involved with providing both physical and emotional care to people. Therefore, the focus of the nurse's concern should be the patient. Items that test your ability to be patient centered tend to explore patient feelings, identify patient preferences, empower the patient, afford the patient choices, or in some other way put emphasis on the patient. Because the patient is the center of the health team, the patient is always the priority.

SAMPLE ITEM 5–11

When assisting a patient who has an above-the-knee amputation to transfer into a chair, the patient starts to cry and says, "I am useless with only one leg." The nurse's best response would be:
(1) "You still have one good leg."
(2) "Losing a leg must be very difficult."
(3) "A prosthesis would make a big difference."
(4) "You'll feel better when you can use crutches."

Option 2 is patient centered. It focuses on the patient's feelings by using the interviewing technique of reflection. Option 1 denies the patient's feelings, and options 3 and 4 provide false reassurance. When a patient's feelings are ignored or minimized, the nurse is not being patient centered. To be patient centered, the nurse should concentrate on the patient's feelings.

SAMPLE ITEM 5–12

An oriented patient complains that he forgets most of the questions he wants to ask when his doctor visits. The nurse should:

(1) Remind him of his next doctor's visit

(2) Offer to stay with him when the doctor visits

(3) Suggest that his family question the doctor for him

(4) Give him paper and a pen to write down his questions

Option 4 is patient centered. It focuses on the patient's ability, fosters independence, and empowers the patient. Option 1 does not address the patient's concern, and options 2 and 3 promote dependence which can lower self-esteem. Avoiding patient concerns and promoting dependence are actions that are not patient centered. To be patient centered, the nurse should encourage self-care.

SAMPLE ITEM 5–13

What should the nurse do first when combing a female patient's hair?

(1) Moisten the hair with tap water

(2) Apply a hair conditioner to the hair

(3) Ask the patient how she prefers to wear her hair

(4) Begin at the roots and comb with long even strokes

Option 3 is patient centered. It allows for choices and supports the person as an individual. Options 1, 2, and 4 do not take into consideration patient preferences. Option 4 is also wrong because combing should begin at the ends of the hair with combing progressively moving toward the roots as tangles are removed. A procedure that is begun prior to determining patient preferences or teaching the patient about the procedure is not patient centered. The Patient's Bill of Rights mandates that the patient has a right to considerate and respectful care and to receive information prior to the start of any procedure and/or treatment.

SAMPLE ITEM 5–14

Mrs. Reid enjoys television programs about animals. After one of these programs Mrs. Reid sadly talks about a cat she once owned. The nurse's initial response should be to:

(1) Tell Mrs. Reid a story about a cat

(2) Hang a picture of a cat in her room

(3) Ask Mrs. Reid to share more about her cat

(4) Obtain a book from the hospital library about cats

    Option 3 is patient centered. It asks an open-ended question that encourages the patient to communicate further. Options 1, 2, and 4 may eventually be done because they take into consideration the patient's interest in cats. However, they should not be the initial actions because they do not focus on the patient and her feelings at this point in time. The nurse is being patient centered when encouraging additional communication and verbalization of feelings and concerns.

Identify Specific Determiners in Options

    A specific determiner is a word or statement that conveys a thought or concept that has no exceptions. Words such as *just, always, never, all, every, none,* and *only* are absolute and easy to identify. They place limits on a statement that would generally be considered correct. Statements that use all-inclusive terms frequently represent broad generalizations that are usually false. Because there are few absolutes in this world, options that contain specific determiners are usually incorrect and can be eliminated.

SAMPLE ITEM 5–15

To best improve circulation during a bath, the nurse should:

(1) Apply soap to the wash cloth

(2) Keep the patient covered

(3) Utilize firm strokes

(4) Use only hot water

    In option 4 the word *only* is a specific determiner. It allows for no exceptions. Hot water could burn the skin and would also be contraindicated for patients with sensitive skin such as children, the elderly, and people with dermatologic problems. Because option 4 allows for no exceptions, it can be eliminated as a viable option.

SAMPLE ITEM 5–16

When providing perineal care for patients, nurses can most appropriately protect themselves from microorganisms by:

(1) Washing their hands prior to giving care

(2) Wearing clean gloves during perineal care

(3) Discarding the contaminated water into the toilet

(4) Encouraging patients to provide all of their own care

    In option 4 the word *all* is a specific determiner. It is a word that obviously includes everything. Expecting patients to provide all of their own care is unreasonable, unrealistic, and could be unsafe. Option 4 can be eliminated. This raises your chances of choosing the correct answer because you have to choose from among only three options rather than four.

SAMPLE ITEM 5–17

Mr. Bond complains that the elastic strap of the oxygen face mask hurts his face. The nurse should:

(1) Explain that it must always stay firmly in place

(2) Replace the face mask with a nasal cannula

(3) Pad the straps with gauze

(4) Adjust the elastic strap

    In option 1 the word *always* is a specific determiner. It is an absolute term that places limits on a statement that might otherwise be true. This option can be eliminated. By deleting option 1, the chances of your selecting the correct answer is 33 rather than 25 percent.

Identify Opposites in Options

    Sometimes an item will contain two options that are opposite to each other. They can be single words that reflect extremes on a continuum, or they can be statements that convey converse messages. When opposites appear in the options, they must be given serious consideration. One of them will be the correct answer, or they both can be eliminated from consideration. When one of the opposites is the correct answer, you are being asked to differentiate between two responses that incorporate extremes of a concept or principle. When the opposites are distractors, they are attempting to divert your attention from the correct answer. If you correctly evaluate opposite options, you can increase your chances of selecting the correct answer to 50 percent because you have reduced the plausible options to two.

SAMPLE ITEM 5–18

The progress of growth and development in all elderly people:

(1) Moves foreward

(2) Becomes slower

(3) Slips backward

(4) Becomes stagnant

Options 1 and 3 are opposites. They need to be carefully considered in relation to each other and then in relation to the other options. These options are the reverse sides of a concept, movement in relation to growth and development. Option 2, although true for some individuals, is not true for *all* elderly people as indicated in the stem. Option 4 can be eliminated because aging is always an advancing process. You now must select between options 1 and 3. Option 3 can be deleted because, as previously stated, aging is an onward process. Option 1 is the correct answer. By focusing on options 1 and 3 and then progressively examining and deleting options 2 and 4, you have systematically scrutinized this item.

SAMPLE ITEM 5–19

The physician orders elastic stockings for a patient. The nurse should put them on:

(1) While the patient is still in bed

(2) When the patient complains of pain

(3) When the patient's feet become edematous

(4) After the patient gets out of bed in the morning

Options 1 and 4 are opposites. Examine these options first. They are contrary to each other in relation to before or after an event, getting out of bed. Now assess options 2 and 3. These options expect the nurse to apply elastic stockings after a problem exists. The purpose of elastic stockings is to foster venous return, thereby preventing edema and discomfort. Options 2 and 3 can be omitted from further consideration. The final selection is between options 1 and 4. You have increased your chances of correctly answering the question from 25 to 50 percent. Because edema occurs when the feet are dependent, elastic stockings should not be applied after the patient gets out of bed. You have arrived at the correct answer, option 1, using a methodical approach.

SAMPLE ITEM 5–20

An arm restraint should be tied to the:

(1) Side rails

(2) Footboard

(3) Headboard

(4) Bed frame

Options 2 and 3 are opposites. Consider these options first in relation to securing a restraint. These options are the opposite ends of a hospital bed. Neither option would be more appropriate than the other. They are probably both distractors. Now examine options 1 and 4. Side rails are movable, and a restraint must be applied to something that is stationary. Now consider option 4. The bed frame is immovable and is independent of the other options. Options 1, 2, and 3 can be eliminated, and option 4 is the correct answer. You have assessed these options in an orderly fashion which has maximized your chances for successfully choosing the correct answer.

SAMPLE ITEM 5–21

In relation to extracellular body fluids, normal saline is:

(1) Hypertonic

(2) Hypotonic

(3) Isotonic

(4) Acidotic

Options 1 and 2 are opposites. Appraise these words in relation to each other and their relationship to body fluids and normal saline. They are extremes in the concentration of solutes. Because normal saline is equal to body fluids in the concentration of solutes, these options are probably distractors. Now examine options 3 and 4. Normal body fluids have a neutral pH (between 7.35 to 7.45). Acidosis, which is referred to in option 4, has a pH below 7.35. Option 4 can be deleted from consideration. By an efficient process of examination and elimination, you have arrived at the correct answer, option 3.

Identify Equally Plausible and Unique Options

Items sometimes contain two or more options that are very similar. It is difficult to choose between them because they are comparable. One option is no better or worse than the other option in relation to the statement presented in the stem. Usually equally plausible options are distractors and can be eliminated from consideration. You have now improved your chances of selecting the correct answer to 50 percent. If you find three equally plausible options when initially examining the options, then the fourth option will probably be different from the others and appear unique. Children's activity books and a popular children's television program present a game based on this concept. Four pictures are presented and the child is asked to pick out the one that is different. Which one of these is not like the others? Which one of these is not the same? For example, the picture contains three types of fruit and one vegetable, and the child is asked to identify which one is different. The correct answer to a test item can sometimes be identified by using this concept of similarities and differences.

SAMPLE ITEM 5–22

To most effectively help meet a patient's basic physical safety and security needs, the nurse should:

(1) Serve adequate food

(2) Provide sufficient fluid

(3) Place the call bell near the patient

(4) Store the patient's valuables in the hospital safe

Options 1 and 2 are similar because they both provide nutrients. They are equally plausible when compared to each other and particularly when assessed in relation to the concepts of safety and security. These options are probably distractors and can be eliminated from consideration. By just having to choose between options 3 and 4, you have raised your chances of correctly answering the question to 50 percent.

SAMPLE ITEM 5–23

To promote circulation when providing a backrub, the nurse should:

(1) Place the patient in the prone position

(2) Use moisturing lotion

(3) Apply baby powder

(4) Knead the skin

Options 2 and 3 utilize substances when performing the backrub. Since no specifics about the patient's adaptations—such as extent of perspiration or dryness of skin—are provided, these two options are comparable. Because equally plausible options are usually distractors, you can delete these options. Now evaluate the remaining options. One of them is probably the correct answer.

SAMPLE ITEM 5–24

Passive range-of-motion exercises are done mainly to:

(1) Increase endurance

(2) Strengthen muscle tone

(3) Maximize muscle atrophy

(4) Prevent loss of mobility

   Options 1, 2, and 3 all improve something: endurance, muscle tone, and atrophy. They are alike. Option 4 is different. It prevents something from happening, loss of mobility. Option 4 is unique when compared to the presentation of the other options, and it should be given careful consideration. Even if you do not know the definition of "atrophy" and do not recognize that the loss of muscle mass should not be maximized, you can still use the test-taking techniques of identifying similar or unique options. Which one of these is not like the others? Which one of these is not the same?

SAMPLE ITEM 5–25

Before performing any patient procedure, the nurse should first plan to:

(1) Shut the door

(2) Wash the hands

(3) Close the curtain

(4) Drape the patient

   Options 1, 3, and 4 are similar in that they all somehow enclose the patient and provide for patient privacy. They are all plausible interventions when providing patient care. It is difficult to choose the most correct answer from among these three options. Option 2 is different. It relates to microbiological safety rather than emotional safety. Since this option is unique in relation to the other options, it should be thoroughly examined in relation to the stem because it is likely to be the correct answer.

Identify Duplicate Facts in Options

   Options sometimes contain two or more facts or statements that are identical or similar. When you can identify one part as being correct, you usually can eliminate at least two options that are distractors. By deleting two distractors, you have increased your chances of selecting the correct answer to 50 percent.

SAMPLE ITEM 5–26

A patient has a vest restraint. While making this patient's occupied bed, what must the nurse do to promote patient safety?

(1) Keep the vest restraint tied and lower both side rails

(2) Keep the vest restraint tied and lower one side rail

(3) Untie the vest restraint and lower both side rails

(4) Untie the vest restraint and lower one side rail

This item is testing two concepts: Should a vest restraint be tied or untied when providing direct care, and should one or both side rails be lowered when providing direct care. If you know the fact that the side rail should be lowered only on the side on which you are working, then you can eliminate options 1 and 3. If you only know the fact that a vest restraint can be untied when the nurse is at the bedside providing direct care, then you can eliminate options 1 and 2. In either case you can eliminate two options as distractors, and you have raised your chances of selecting the correct answer from 25 to 50 percent.

SAMPLE ITEM 5–27

The physician orders a 2-gram sodium diet. Which of the following groups of nutrients would be most appropriate for this diet?

(1) Fruit, vegetables, and bread

(2) Hamburger, onions, and ketchup

(3) Hot dogs, mustard, and pickles

(4) Luncheon meats, rolls, and vegetables

This item is testing knowledge about the sodium content of foods. If you recognize that hot dogs and luncheon meats are both processed foods which are high in sodium, then you can eliminate options 3 and 4. If you recognize that ketchup and mustard are both condiments which are high in sodium, then you can delete options 2 and 3. By knowing either fact, you can reduce the final selection to between two options. The similarities between these options are more obscure than if the parts were identical, but the technique of identifying duplicate facts in options can still be used.

SAMPLE ITEM 5–28

When monitoring a patient who is at risk for hemorrhage, the nurse should assess the patient for:

(1) Warm dry skin, hypotension, bounding pulse

(2) Hypertension, bounding pulse, cold clammy skin

(3) Weak thready pulse, hypertension, warm dry skin

(4) Hypotension, cold clammy skin, weak thready pulse

This item is testing your knowledge about patient adaptations associated with hemorrhage. Three patient adaptations are presented: the condition of the skin, the blood pressure, and the characteristic of the pulse. Even if you know only one of these facts about hemorrhage, you can reduce your final selection to between two options. If you know that hypotension is associated with hemorrhage, then you can eliminate options 2 and 3. If you know that cold clammy skin is related to hemorrhage, then you can delete options 1 and 3. If you know that a weak thready pulse is associated with hemorrhage, then you can eliminate options 1 and 2. If you know only one or two of the facts presented, you can maximize the information you do possess in answering this type of item. Options that have three parts work to your advantage if you utilize the technique of identifying duplicate facts in options.

Identify Options That Deny Patient Feelings, Concerns, and Needs

Because nurses are human, caring, and primarily want their patients to get well, they often assume the roles of deliverer, champion, protector, or savior. However, by inappropriately adopting these roles, nurses often diminish patient concerns, provide false reassurance, and/or cut off further patient communication. To be a patient advocate, the nurse cannot always be a Pollyanna. Pollyanna was a person of irrepressible optimism who found good in everything, the heroine of stories by Eleanor Hodgman Porter. Sometimes nurses must focus on the negative rather than the positive, acknowledge that everything may not have the desired outcome, and recognize patient feelings as a priority. Options that imply everything will be all right, deny patient feelings, change the subject raised by the patient, encourage the patient to be cheerful, or abdicate nursing responsibility to other members of the health team are usually distractors and can be eliminated from consideration.

SAMPLE ITEM 5–29

The night before surgery for a hysterectomy, the patient says to the nurse, "I am worried that I might die tomorrow." The nurse's best response would be:

(1) "It is really routine surgery."
(2) "Have you told your doctor about this?"
(3) "The thought of dying can be frightening."
(4) "Most people who have this surgery survive."

Options 1 and 4 dispute the patient's concerns because the nurse's messages imply that there is nothing to worry about; the surgery is routine and most patients survive. In option 2 the nurse avoids the opportunity to encourage a further discussion of the patient's feelings and surrenders this responsibility to the physician. After collecting more information, the nurse may inform the physician of the patient's concern about death. Options 1, 2, and 4 deny the patient's feelings and can be eliminated because they are distractors. Option 3 is the correct answer because it encourages the patient to focus on the expressed feelings about death.

SAMPLE ITEM 5–30

Following surgery the patient complains of mild incisional pain while performing deep-breathing and coughing exercises. The nurse's best response would be:

(1) "Each day it will hurt less and less."
(2) "This is an expected response after surgery."
(3) "With a pillow apply pressure against the incision."
(4) "I will get the pain medication the physician ordered."

Option 1 is a Pollyanna-like response that provides false reassurance. The nurse does not know that the pain will get less and less for this patient. Option 1 can be deleted from consideration. Although option 2 is a true statement, it cuts off communication because it diminishes the patient's concern and does not explore a solution for minimizing the pain. Option 2 can be eliminated as as distractor. You now must choose between options 3 and 4. The stem indicates that the patient has pain when coughing; the pain is not continuous. Option 4 can be deleted because it would be inappropriate to administer an analgesic at this time. The correct answer is option 3 because it recognizes the pain and offers an intervention to help relieve the discomfort. Each time you can eliminate an option that denies a patient's feelings, you raise your chances of selecting the correct answer.

SAMPLE ITEM 5–31

An elderly woman with a right-sided hemiplegia and tears in her eyes sadly states, "I used to brush my hair a 100 strokes a day and now I have to rely on others to do it." The nurse's initial response should be:

(1) "It must be hard not to be able to do things for yourself."

(2) "Let me brush your hair a 100 strokes, and then I'll help you with breakfast."

(3) "With physical therapy you will be able to brush your own hair again some day."

(4) "That's true, but there are lots of other things you are capable of doing for yourself."

Option 2 changes the subject and cuts off communication. Option 3 is a Pollyanna-like response because it implies that everything will eventually be all right. Option 4 initially accepts the patient's statement but then attempts to refocus the patient on the positive before exploring the negative. Options 2, 3, and 4 in one way or another deny the patient's feelings, concerns, and/or needs. The correct answer is option 1 because it is an open-ended statement that focuses on the patient's feelings.

Utilize Multiple Test-Taking Techniques

You have just been introduced to a variety of test-taking techniques. As you practice applying each of these techniques to test items, you will become more skillful at being test-wise. As you become more proficient at applying test-taking techniques, you can further maximize success in choosing the correct option if you utilize more than one test-taking technique within an item.

to page 102

SAMPLE ITEM 5–32

Mr. Lance's nursing care plan indicates that passive range-of-motion (PROM) exercises of the right leg are to be done every 2 hours while awake. The nurse should:

(1) Move the patient's leg through PROM when indicated

(2) Demonstrate how to perform PROM exercises

(3) Explain that all patients do PROM by themselves

(4) Take the patient to physical therapy for PROM exercises

　　Option 3 includes the specific determiner *all* and should be carefully evaluated. Some patients are able to perform PROM exercises themselves (e.g., a patient with a hemiplegia can perform PROM on the affected arm and hand with the extremity that is unaffected) while some patients are unable to perform PROM (e.g., a patient with quadriplegia). Because some patients cannot perform PROM exercises, there are exceptions to the statement in option 3. This option can be deleted from consideration by using the technique Identify Specific Determiners in Options. Option 4 abdicates responsibility for care that the nurse is educated and licensed to provide. This option can be eliminated from consideration by using the technique Identify Options That Deny Patient Feelings, Concerns, and/or Needs. By utilizing two test-taking techniques, you have eliminated options 3 and 4, reduced the number of options to two, and increased your chances of selecting the correct answer to 50 percent.

SAMPLE ITEM 5–33

Patient adaptations that are both unexpected in response to the general adaptation syndrome are:

(1) Dilated pupils and bradycardia

(2) Mental alertness and tachycardia

(3) Decreased blood glucose and bradycardia

(4) Increased blood glucose and tachycardia

　　By carefully reading the stem, you should identify that the word "unexpected" is a significant word in this item. You have just used the test-taking technique Identify Key Words in the Stem That Indicate Negative Polarity. If you know that tachycardia is associated with the general adaptation syndrome, you can eliminate options 2 and 4. This utilizes the test-taking technique Identify Duplicate Facts in Options. If you recognize that options 3 and 4 are opposites, you should give these options particular consideration. By seriously considering these options, you are using the test-taking technique Identify Opposites in Options. A variety of test-taking techniques can be applied to analyze and answer this item.

SAMPLE ITEM 5–34

When the nurse administers a backrub to reduce the physical discomfort of a backache, the nurse is meeting a patient's:

(1) Safety needs

(2) Security needs

(3) Self-esteem needs

(4) Physiological needs

By thoughtfully reading the stem you should identify that the important words are *reduce the physical discomfort of a backache.* When reviewing the options, you should recognize that the word "physiological" in option 4 is closely related to the word "physical" in the stem. Option 4 should be given serious consideration. Options 1 and 2 present the words "safety" and "security." They are comparable, and choosing between them would be difficult. They probably are distractors. This utilizes the test-taking technique Identify Equally Plausible and/or Unique Options. The use of multiple test-taking techniques in an item can facilitate the deletion of distractors and the selection of the correct answer.

GENERAL TEST-TAKING TECHNIQUES

A general test-taking technique is a strategy that is utilized to conquer the challenge of an examination. To be in command of the situation, you must be able to manage your internal and external domains. The test-taker who approaches a test with physical, mental, and emotional authority is in a better position to regulate the testing situation, rather than have the testing situation dominate.

Follow Your Regular Routine the Night Before a Test

Follow your normal routine the night before a test. This is not the time to make changes that may disrupt your equilibrium. If you do not normally eat pepperoni pizza, exercise, or study until 2 AM, do not start now. Go to bed at your usual time. Avoid the temptation to have an all-night cram session. Studies have demonstrated that sleep deprivation decreases reaction times and cognitive skills. An adequate night's sleep is necessary to produce a rested mind and body that provide the physical and emotional energy required to maximize performance on an examination.

Arrive on Time for the Examination

Plan your schedule so that you arrive at the testing site approximately 15 to 30 minutes early. Arrange extra time for unexpected events associated with traveling. There may be a traffic jam, a road may have a detour, the car may not start, the train may be late, the bus could break down, or you may have to park in the farthest lot from the testing site. If the location of the testing site or classroom is unfamiliar to you, it would be wise to take a practice run and locate the room. On the day of the examination you want to avoid getting lost.

By arriving early, you have an opportunity to visit the restroom, survey the situation, and collect your thoughts. Because anxiety is associated with an autonomic nervous system response, you may have urgency, frequency, or increased intestinal peristalsis. Visit the restroom before the test to avoid utilizing testing time to meet physical needs. The test may or may not be administered in the room in which the content is taught. Arriving early allows you to survey the situation and become more comfortable in the testing environment. Decide where you want to sit if seats are not assigned. Students have preferences such as sitting by a window, being in the back of the room, or surrounding themselves with friends. Selecting your own seat allows you to manipulate one aspect of your environment. In addition, this time before the test provides you with an opportunity to collect your thoughts. You may desire to review content on a flash card, perform relaxation exercises, or reinforce your positive mental attitude. However, avoid comparing notes with other students. They may have inaccurate information or be anxious. Remember anxiety is contagious. If you are the type who is readily affected by the anxiety of other people, evade these people until after the test.

Bring the Appropriate Tools

To perform a task, you need adequate tools. Pens, pencils, and an eraser are essential. A pen is usually required to complete the identifying information on the answer sheet. A pencil is usually necessary to record your answers on the answer sheet if it is a computer answer form. Use number 2 pencils because they have soft lead that facilitate the computer scoring of the answer sheet. Bring at least two pens and two or more pencils. Backup equipment is advisable because ink can run out and points can break. Sharpen all your pencils and/or bring a small, self-contained pencil sharpener if you prefer to work with a sharp point on your pencil. Have at least one eraser. You may decide to change an answer or need to erase extraneous marks that you make on the question book or the answer sheet. A watch is also a necessary tool for every test. Some proctors will announce time frames as the test progresses and others will not. Bringing your own watch provides you with a sense of independence and control. Depending on your individual needs, other tools might include eyeglasses, a hearing aid, or a calculator. Assemble all your equipment the night before the test, and be sure to take them with you to the testing site.

Understand All the Directions for the Test Before Starting

It is essential to understand the instructions before beginning the test. On some tests you are responsible for independently reading the instructions while on others the proctor verbally announces the instructions. However, more often than not you will have a written copy of the instructions while the proctor reads them aloud. In this instance do not read ahead of the proctor. The proctor may elaborate on the written instructions, and you do not want to miss any of the additional directions. If you do not understand a particular part of the instructions, immediately request that the proctor explain them again. You must completely understand the instructions before beginning the examination.

Manage the Allotted Time to Your Advantage

All tests have a time limit. Some tests have severe time restrictions in which most test-takers do not complete all the questions on the examination. These are known as "speed tests." Other tests have a generous time frame in which the majority of test-takers have ample time to answer every question on the examination. These are known as "power tests." The purpose of tests in nursing is to identify how much information the test-taker possesses about the nursing care of people. Most nursing examinations are power tests. Regardless of the type of test, you must utilize your time well.

To manage your time on an examination, you must determine how much time you have to answer each item while leaving some time for review at the end of the testing period. To ascertain how much time you should allot for each item, divide the total time you have for the test by the number of items on the test. For example, if you have 90 minutes to take a test that has 50 items, divide 90 by 50. This allots 1 minute and 48 seconds for each item. If you actually allot 1½ minutes per item, you will leave 15 minutes for a final review. Be aware of the time as you progress through a test. If you determine that you have approximately 1½ minutes for each question, then by the time you have completed 10 items, 15 minutes should have passed. Pace yourself so that you do not spend more than 1½ minutes on an item if possible. If you answer an item in less than 1½ minutes, then you can utilize the excess time for another item that may take slightly longer than 1½ minutes or add this time to the end for review. The allocation of time for test completion depends on the complexity of the content, the difficulty of the reading level, and the number of options presented in the items. Nursing examinations generally allot 1 minute per item when there are four options.

Utilize all the time allocated for the examination. The test constructors calculated that the time parameters for the test were appropriate for a thoughtful review of the items. Read the items slowly and carefully. If you process items too quickly, you may overlook important words, become careless, or arrive at impulsive conclusions. Work at your own pace. Do not be influenced by the actions of other test-takers. If other test-takers complete the examination early, ignore them and do not become concerned. Just because they finish early does not indicate that they will score well on the test. They may be imprudent speed demons. A cautious, discriminating, and judicious approach is to your advantage. Be your own person, and remember that time can be your ally rather than your adversary.

Concentrate on the Simple Before the Complex

Answer the easy questions before the difficult questions. This utilizes the basic teaching-learning principle of moving from the simple to the complex. By doing this, you can maximize your use of time and maintain a positive mental attitude. Begin answering questions. When you confront a difficult item, and you have already used your allotted time to answer it, and you still do not know the answer, then skip over this item and move on to the next one. Make a notation on scrap paper, next to the item in the question booklet, and/or next to the number of the skipped item on the answer sheet so that you can return to this item later in the test. Making a mark on the answer sheet should prevent you from making the error of recording the next answer in the previous item's location on the answer sheet. These and any other extraneous marks must be erased from the answer sheet before handing it in to the proctor. Extraneous marks confuse the computer, and you will probably lose credit because it will be scored as an incorrect answer. When you reach the end of the test, return to those items that you reserved for the end. You should have more time to spend on these items, and you may have accessed information from other items that can assist you in answering these questions. Concentrating on the simple before the complex permits you to answer the maximum number of items in the time allocated for the examination.

Make Educated Guesses

An educated guess occurs when you select an option without knowing for certain that it is actually the correct answer. The selection is based on partial knowledge. When you reduce the final selection to two options, it is usually to your advantage to reassess these options in context of the knowledge you do possess and make an educated guess. Making a wild guess by flipping a coin or choosing your favorite number should depend on whether or not the test has a penalty for guessing.

Some examinations assign credit when you select a correct answer and do not allocate credit when you select one of the distractors. The instructions for these examinations may state in the directions that only correct answers will receive credit, you should answer every question, you should not leave any blanks, or that there are no penalties for guessing. In these tests it is to your advantage to answer every question. First, select answers based on knowledge. If you are unsure of the correct answer, reduce the number of options and then make an educated guess. If you have absolutely no idea what the answer can be, then make a wild guess because you will not be penalized for a wrong answer.

Some tests will assign credit when you select a correct answer and will subtract credit when you select a distractor. The instructions for these examinations may inform you not to guess, that credit will be subtracted for incorrect answers, or there is a penalty for guessing. In these tests a statistical manipulation is performed to mathematically limit the advantage of guessing. When taking these tests, it is still to your advantage to make an educated guess if through knowledge you can reduce your final selection to two options. However, wild guessing is not to your advantage because you are penalized for guessing.

Maintain a Positive Mental Attitude

It is important that you foster a positive mental attitude and a sense of relaxation. A little apprehension can be motivating, but when it rises too much, it can interfere with your attention, concentration, and problem-solving ability. Utilize positive techniques you have practiced and that work for you to enhance relaxation and a positive mental attitude. For example, feel in control by skipping the difficult questions; enhance relaxation by employing diaphragmatic breathing for several deep breaths, rotating your shoulders, or flexing and hyperextending your head; foster a positive mental attitude by telling yourself, "I am prepared to do this well!" or "I know I have studied hard and I will be successful!"

Check Your Answers and Answer Sheet

Most examinations incorporate time at the end of the testing period for review. Reassess your answers, particularly for those items in which you made an educated guess. Subsequent questions may contain content that is helpful to answering a previous question, you may access information you did not remember originally, or you may be less anxious and are able to assess the question with more objectivity. Be aware of your success in changing answers on previous tests. Every time you review a test, evaluate your accuracy in changing answers. Keep score of how many answers you change from wrong to right and how many you change from right to wrong. If the number of items you changed from wrong to right is greater than the number of items you changed from right to wrong, then it would probably be to your advantage to change answers you ultimately believe you answered incorrectly. On the other hand, if you change more answers from right to wrong, then you should avoid changing your answers unless you are positive that your second choice is the correct choice. Make sure that you have answered every question, especially on tests that do not penalize for guessing.

Review your answer sheet for accuracy. Computer-scored tests usually utilize separate answer sheets in which each item has numbers or letters that represent the corresponding responses to each item in the test. Make sure that every mark is within the lines, heavy and full, and in the appropriate space. Erase any extraneous marks on the answer sheet. Additional pencil marks, inadequately erased answers, and marks outside the lines will confuse the computer and alter your score. An effective and thorough review should leave you with a feeling of control and a sense of closure at the end of the examination.

ANSWERS AND RATIONALES FOR SAMPLE ITEMS IN CHAPTER 5

An asterisk (*) is in front of the rationale that explains the correct answer.

5–1   (1) Used linens may be contaminated with body secretions; wearing gloves is part of universal precautions.

    * (2) These linens are considered soiled, and if returned, they would contaminate the linen room.

    (3) This is an acceptable practice if the sheet is not wet or soiled.

    (4) This is an acceptable practice; the entire bed is washed with a disinfectant between patients.

5–2   (1) Stewed fruit is low in sodium.

    * (2) Luncheon meats are generally processed with large amounts of sodium.

    (3) Whole-grain cereal is low in sodium.

    (4) Green leafy vegetables are low in sodium.

5–3   (1) Kneading the skin increases circulation and should be part of a backrub unless contraindicated.

    (2) Excess lotion can be an irritant to the skin and should be removed.

    (3) This is soothing and relieves muscle tension; this action is based on the gate control theory of pain relief.

    * (4) This action should be avoided because it can cause unnecessary pressure over bony prominences; strokes should massage muscle groups, not vertebrae.

5–4 * (1) Ointments and jellies have an oil base that provides a barrier; they also hold in moisture which prevents drying and cracking of skin.

    (2) Although these pads are often used for patients who are incontinent, they tend to hold urine and feces against the skin promoting maceration and skin breakdown.

(3) Although this is often used, when excessive amounts are mixed with urine and perspiration, it results in a paste that promotes the growth of microorganisms, and it can be an irritant.

(4) Same as #3.

5–5 * (1) This should be done first. It is essential that the specific type of enema ordered be given; enemas have different solutions, volumes, and purposes.

(2) This is done after the type of enema is verified; each type of enema has different requirements.

(3) This should be done once all the equipment and the patient are prepared and ready.

(4) This action is implemented once the nurse verifies the type of enema ordered; the nurse's explanation depends on the type of enema being administered.

5–6   (1) This would be done later; the nurse's first action is to support the patient.

(2) Same as #1.

(3) Same as #1.

  * (4) The patient is the priority at this time; once the patient is protected and safe, the actions of the abusive nurse must be addressed.

5–7   (1) This is a demeaning response and does not answer the patient's question.

(2) Not responding would make the patient more upset; the patient has a right to know who is providing care.

(3) This denies the patient's concern and does not answer the question.

  * (4) This answers the question, which meets the patient's right to know; it is also a respectful response.

5–8   (1) Food is only one aspect of a society and its culture; the primary purpose of food is to meet physiological needs.

(2) Although alcohol meets some people's psychological needs and is served in social situations, it is not the factor that most influences psychosocial development.

  * (3) A person's cultural environment, which includes the family and the community, has the most impact on psychosocial development.

(4) Although genetics has been identified by some theorists to be a factor related to personality and behavior, it is not the most influential factor in psychosocial development.

5–9 * (1) This encourages independence, which increases self-esteem.

(2) This would meet the patient's needs for love and belonging, not self-esteem.

(3) When a person is dependent on another, such dependency often lowers self-esteem.

(4) Same as #3.

5–10 (1) This action supports self-esteem needs, not physical needs.

(2) This action meets safety needs, not physical needs.

  * (3) This meets a patient's basic physiological need to be clean.

(4) Vital signs are not a physiological need, but an assessment done by the nurse to determine needs.

5–11 (1) This denies the patient's feelings.

  * (2) This focuses on the patient's feelings by the use of reflection.

(3) This is false reassurance.

(4) Same as #3.

5–12   (1) This does not address the patient's concern; the patient forgets the questions to be asked, not when the physician will visit.

        (2) This may foster feelings of dependence and could violate the patient's privacy if the questions to be asked are personal.

        (3) Same as #2.

    * (4) This promotes independence, self-esteem, and privacy.

5–13   (1) This may be done after obtaining the patient's permission.

        (2) Same as #1.

   * (3) This promotes individualized care by allowing personal choices.

        (4) This is unsafe; combing should begin at the ends and progressively move toward the roots as tangles are removed.

5–14   (1) Although this may eventually be done, the primary intervention should be exploring the patient's feelings.

        (2) Same as #1.

    * (3) This is an open-ended question that encourages verbalization of feelings.

        (4) Same as #1.

5–15   (1) Soap lowers the surface tension of water, which promotes cleaning, not circulation.

        (2) This does not improve local circulation; it only prevents chilling.

   * (3) Pressure and friction produce local heat, which dilates blood vessels, improving circulation.

        (4) Hot water can damage delicate tissue and should be avoided; bath water should be between 110 and 115°F.

5–16   (1) This protects the patient from the nurse.

   * (2) Gloves are a barrier against body secretions and are used with universal precautions.

        (3) This is unsafe; the nurse is still exposed to body secretions if not wearing gloves.

        (4) This is unreasonable and inappropriate; some patients need assistance with meeting their needs.

5–17   (1) Straps and a mask that are firm against the skin can cause tissue trauma; the elastic straps can be adjusted for comfort while keeping the edges of the mask gently against the skin.

        (2) This method of oxygen delivery requires a physician's order.

        (3) Although this might be done, it does not address the tightness of the mask against the skin of the face.

    * (4) Loosening the elastic straps will reduce the pressure of the mask against the face.

5–18 * (1) Aging, from conception to death, advances and moves onward.

        (2) Although this may be true for some elderly, it is not true for all.

        (3) This is untrue; aging is progressive and does not move backward.

        (4) Same as #2.

5–19 * (1) Dependent edema is minimal while the feet are still elevated; elastic stockings should be applied before the legs are moved to a dependent position.

        (2) The purpose of elastic stockings is to promote venous return, not reduce pain.

(3) This would cause tissue trauma because of the presence of fluid in the interstitial compartment; they are applied to prevent edema.

(4) Elastic stockings should be applied before the feet are moved to a dependent position.

5-20 (1) This is unsafe; they do not provide a stable base of support. Injury can occur when the rails are inadvertently lowered before the straps are removed.

(2) This would require an excessively long strap in which the patient's legs could get entangled.

(3) This could result in an uncomfortable line of pull with the arm above the head.

* (4) This is a stable base of support and is beyond the patient's reach.

5-21 (1) A solution is hypertonic when the total electrolyte content is 375 mEq/L or greater.

(2) A solution is hypotonic when the total electrolyte content is below 250 mEq/L.

* (3) A solution is isotonic when the total electrolyte content is approximately 310 mEq/L; normal saline (sodium chloride) is isotonic.

(4) This refers to excessive levels of hydrogen ions in the blood affecting pH values.

5-22 (1) Nutrients, such as food and fluids, meet basic physiological needs.

(2) Same as #1.

* (3) Being able to summon help when needed provides a sense of security for the patient.

(4) This provides for emotional safety.

5-23 (1) This exposes the entire area to permit a thorough backrub; it does not promote circulation.

(2) This moisturizes the skin and makes it supple; it does not promote circulation.

(3) Although this is often used for backrubs to permit the hands to slide against the skin, it should not be used for patients who perspire because it can cause a pastelike substance that promotes skin breakdown.

* (4) Kneading causes friction and pressure against the skin that promotes localized heat, precipitates vessel dilation, and improves circulation.

5-24 (1) Active range of motion, not passive range of motion, can increase endurance.

(2) Active range of motion can strengthen muscle tone, not passive range of motion.

(3) Passive range of motion is done to prevent muscle shortening resulting in contractures. Atrophy is the loss of muscle mass due to lack of muscle contraction, not lack of joint mobility.

* (4) Passive range-of-motion exercises prevent shortening of muscles, ligaments, and tendons, which causes a joint to become fixed in one position.

5-25 (1) This provides for privacy and prevents drafts, but if the nurse's hands are not clean, they will contaminate the door.

* (2) Between patients and before providing care, the nurse must wash the hands to remove dirt and microorganisms; otherwise, equipment and the patient will be affected by cross-contamination. Medical asepsis is a priority.

(3) This provides for privacy and prevents drafts, but if the nurse's hands are not clean, they will contaminate the curtain.

(4) This provides for privacy and prevents evaporation and chilling, but if the nurse's hands are not clean, they will contaminate the linen and patient.

5–26   (1) Both actions could injure the patient; the patient could fall out of bed on the side opposite to the nurse; moving a patient while restrained exerts stress on the musculoskeletal systems.

     (2) This is unsafe; moving a patient while restrained could injure the patient.

     (3) This is unsafe; lowering the side rail on the side opposite to which the nurse is working could result in the patient's falling out of bed.

   * (4) Untying a restraint permits free movement, which limits stress on the musculoskeletal systems. Lowering one side rail allows the nurse to provide direct care. Keeping the side rail raised on the side opposite to which the nurse is working provides a barrier to prevent falling out of bed.

5–27 * (1) These foods contain the least amount of sodium as compared to the other options.

     (2) Ketchup is high in sodium and should be avoided.

     (3) These all contain a high level of sodium and should be avoided.

     (4) Luncheon meats are processed foods that contain a high level of sodium and should be avoided.

5–28   (1) With hemorrhage the skin would be cold and clammy, not warm and dry, and the pulse would be weak and thready, not bounding.

     (2) Because of the reduced blood volume associated with hemorrhage, the blood pressure would be decreased, not increased, and the pulse would be weak and thready, not bounding.

     (3) With hemorrhage the blood pressure would be decreased, not increased, and the skin would be cold and clammy, not warm and dry.

   * (4) Because of the decreased blood volume associated with hemorrhage, there would be a reduced blood pressure and weak thready pulse; because of the autonomic nervous system response and the constriction of peripheral blood vessels, the skin would be cold and clammy.

5–29   (1) This denies the patient's feelings about death and cuts off further communication.

     (2) This abdicates the responsibility of the nurse to explore the patients's feelings to the physician; it cuts off communication and does not meet the patient's immediate need to discuss fears of death.

   * (3) This uses reflective technique because it focuses on the underlying feeling expressed in the patient's statement.

     (4) Same as #1.

5–30   (1) This is a Pollyanna-like response that provides false reassurance.

     (2) Although this is a true statement, it cuts off communication and does not present an intervention to help limit the discomfort.

   * (3) This recognizes the pain and offers an intervention to help limit the discomfort.

     (4) This would be inappropriate at this time; analgesics should be administered if the pain is acute or continues after the exercises are completed.

5–31 * (1) This identifies the patient's concern and offers an opportunity to further discuss the topic.

     (2) This reinforces feelings of dependence, changes the subject, and cuts off communication.

(3) This is a Pollyanna-like response that provides false reassurance; the patient may never be able to brush her own hair.

(4) Once the patient's present feelings are explored, then pointing out the patient's abilities would be appropriate.

5–32 * (1) This activity is within the role of the nurse, provides for continuity of care, and meets the patient's need to prevent contractures.

(2) PROM exercises of a leg cannot be performed independently; this is appropriate for active range-of-motion exercises.

(3) Some patients are not capable of performing PROM exercises depending on the strength of the unaffected extremity and their physical, mental, and/or emotional status.

(4) This abdicates the nurse's responsibility to other members of the health team.

5–33 (1) Tachycardia, not bradycardia, is associated with the general adaptation syndrome (GAS); dilated pupils are expected.

(2) Both these adaptations are expected autonomic nervous system responses that occur during the alarm stage of the GAS.

* (3) During the alarm stage of the GAS, both the blood glucose level and heart rate increase, not decrease.

(4) Same as #2.

5–34 (1) Safety and security needs, the second level of needs according to Maslow, are met when the patient is protected from harm.

(2) Same as #1.

(3) Self-esteem needs are met when the patient is treated with dignity and respect.

* (4) Being free from pain or discomfort is a basic physiological need; a backrub improves local circulation, reduces muscle tension, and limits pain.

6 Fundamentals of Nursing Practice Tests

INTRODUCTION TO PRACTICE TESTS

Three practice tests have been provided so you can measure your knowledge of nursing content and test-taking skills for the purpose of comparison over time. Each test has been designed to test items with comparable content, in similar proportions to those you may find on a fundamentals of nursing examination, and with a similar degree of difficulty. Utilize these tests in a planned way. Do not take them haphazardly. Take Practice Test A before reading any of the chapters in this book. This will assess your knowledge of the fundamentals of nursing content and your ability to take a test. This test functions as a pretest, and your score will provide a baseline for future comparison. Carefully read Chapters 1 through 5 at your own pace. Once you complete reading these chapters, take Practice Test B. This will provide an interim score regarding your test-taking performance. Now study the practice questions in Chapter 7. The questions in Chapter 7 are grouped within content areas. It would be most beneficial to study these content areas after you have covered this content in your curriculum. Take Test C after you have completed Chapter 7. This final test will serve as a post-test. Hopefully you should improve your score each time you take a subsequent practice test.

Simulated testing is designed to demonstrate growth and motivate you to continue with your efforts to succeed in testing situations. The order in which you take the tests does not matter. You can choose to take Practice Test C first and then B and A. The three tests have been designed so that the tests are equal in their level of difficulty. The average score for each test is approximately 76 percent. This was determined by a statistical analysis of field testing conducted with fundamental nursing students from a variety of nursing schools from across the country. If your score is greater than 76 percent on any of the tests, you will have scored higher than the average fundamental nursing student that participated in the field testing. If your score is less than 76 percent, you will have scored lower than the average fundamental nursing student that participated in the field testing.

When self-administering a practice test, set aside 40 minutes of uninterrupted time. To simulate a testing environment, you must sit at a table and select a time when you will not be disturbed. You are allotted 40 minutes to take one practice test. If you divide 40 minutes by 30 questions, you have approximately 1⅓ minutes to consider each question. To leave 10 minutes at the end of the examination for review, permit yourself 1 minute to answer each question. If you spend less than 1 minute on a question, you can utilize this time for the questions you find more difficult or add it to the time you have reserved for your review at the end of the test. Use the full 40 minutes to complete each practice test.

When taking a practice test, use the answer sheets provided at the end of the book. To record your answers, use a number 2 pencil because the lead is soft enough to easily fill the spaces provided on the answer sheet. Carefully darken the enclosed space on the answer sheet that corresponds to the number of the question on the test. This is particularly relevant if you should skip over an item that is difficult. When you come across an item that you find difficult, skip it and move on to the next item. However, when you record your next answer ensure that you darken the appropriate place on the answer sheet. Students have been known to score poorly on an important test because they inadvertently placed an answer on the wrong line causing each subsequent answer to be incorrectly recorded. Answer every question. If you do not know the answer to a question, attempt to eliminate as many options as you can using test-taking skills and then make an educated guess.

After you complete a practice test, review the correct answer and rationales for the correct and incorrect options. Analyze the reasons you may have selected a distractor instead of the correct answer. Ask yourself, "Was I careless?" "Did I lack knowledge about the content?" "Did I miss an important word in the stem?" "Did I quickly jump to the wrong conclusion?" "Did I read into the question and make it more complicated?" or "Did I misunderstand what the question was asking?" It is important to identify why you answer an item incorrectly so that you can implement some corrective action to improve your score the next time. As you review the practice test, make notes referring to content that you answered incorrectly. If you had difficulty answering questions related to patient assessments or content concerning hygiene, then you should direct your future study toward these areas of concern. Also analyze the results of every item in which you changed your initial answer. If when you change an answer you invariably get the item correct, you might continue to profit from changing your answers on succeeding tests. If when you change an answer you consistently get the item wrong, it may be to your advantage not to change your answers on subsequent tests. However, determine what it was that caused you to change your initial choice to the correct or incorrect answer. If you can identify patterns of errors in test taking, you may be able to institute strategies to eliminate them on future examinations. Practice tests are learning experiences because they permit the application of test-taking strategies, reinforce information you understand, identify content areas that need to be emphasized in future study, and build your test-taking endurance.

PRACTICE TEST A

1. Mrs. Green has just been informed that she will be transferred to a nursing home because her son is unable to care for her at home. While providing a bed bath, Mrs.

Green yells at the nurse, "You don't know what you are doing." The nurse's *best* reaction would be to:
(1) Request that another nurse take care of Mrs. Green
(2) Accept the behavior and not take it personally
(3) Discontinue the bath and resume it later
(4) Explain that she is getting good care

2. A patient is wearing bilateral mitt restraints. The nurse should release the restraints and massage and exercise the hands and wrists every:
(1) Hour
(2) Shift
(3) 2 hours
(4) 4 hours

3. A patient is found with stool smeared on his body, the linens, and the bed rails. The initial goal should be that the resident will:
(1) Be clean and dry
(2) Become continent
(3) Call for the bedpan
(4) Stop smearing stool

4. The best action for the nurse to take to prevent the patient from falling out of bed when using a bedpan should be to:
(1) Raise the side rails on both sides of the bed
(2) Place an overbed table in front of the patient
(3) Reposition the patient to a semi-Fowler's position
(4) Lower the height of the bed to its lowest position

5. Mrs. Jones, who is often short of breath, is afraid to be left alone in her room. To help reduce her fear, the nurse should:
(1) Position her in a wheelchair near the nurses' station
(2) Encourage her to become friends with her roommate
(3) Stay with her as much as possible
(4) Answer her call bell immediately

6. A patient has bilateral wrist restraints. To provide adequate fluid intake, the nurse should:
(1) Encourage extra fluids at each meal
(2) Serve fluids frequently between meals
(3) Position a glass of water within reach
(4) Provide a long straw to encourage drinking

7. Obese patients often have serious difficulty breathing when positioned in the:
(1) Supine position
(2) Contour position
(3) Orthopneic position
(4) Semi-Fowler's position

8. Which of the following facts about ambulation is most important to document in the patient's medical record?
(1) When the patient is ambulated
(2) Where the patient is ambulated
(3) The patient's response to ambulation
(4) The length of time it took to ambulate the patient

9. To provide the most therapeutic communication with a patient, the nurse should:
(1) Utilize direct questions
(2) Teach about self-care

    (3) Ask direct questions
    (4) Listen attentively

10. A physical reaction to moderate pain is:
    (1) Crying
    (2) Moaning
    (3) Increased heart rate
    (4) Complaints of suffering

11. Which of the following is an accurate statement?
    (1) Daily baths are necessary for homeostasis
    (2) Bathing decreases pathogens on the skin
    (3) A bath is ineffective without soap
    (4) Patients want to be clean and neat

12. The nurse makes a work assignment for the nursing assistant at the beginning of the shift. An acceptable expectation of the nurse is that the nursing assistant will:
    (1) Complete everything that has been assigned
    (2) Be friendly with other health team members
    (3) Work with minimal supervision by the nurse
    (4) Perform within the limits of the nursing assistant role

13. Mr. Sing is cognitively impaired and confused. When assisting Mr. Sing with his meal, the nurse should say:
    (1) "What would you like to eat first?"
    (2) "It is good for you to eat all your food."
    (3) "This is your meat. Please eat your meat."
    (4) "If you finish your meat, then you can have dessert."

14. Which of the following patients would require a rectal temperature rather than an oral temperature?
    (1) A woman with no teeth
    (2) A man receiving oxygen
    (3) An 8-year-old child
    (4) An elderly man with dentures

15. A patient with an indwelling urinary catheter (Foley) is to be transferred to a wheelchair. To prevent reflux of urine into the bladder, the nurse should plan to:
    (1) Attach the bag to the arm of the wheelchair
    (2) Place it on the floor under the wheelchair
    (3) Place the bag in the patient's lap
    (4) Hang it on the chair below the patient's hip

16. The patient at the highest risk for developing a decubitus ulcer would be a patient with:
    (1) Paraplegia
    (2) Hypotension
    (3) Memory loss
    (4) Heart failure

17. The most effective method to prevent the spread of microorganisms to all the patients in a hospital is:
    (1) Medical asepsis
    (2) Surgical asepsis
    (3) Isolation precautions
    (4) The use of antibiotics

18. After performing an IM injection, a drop of blood appears at the injection site. The nurse should:
    (1) Massage the area gently
    (2) Take the patient's vital signs

(3) Apply pressure with the antiseptic swab
(4) Document this reaction in the nurse's notes

19. A patient is ordered to be on intake and output. Which of the following foods should be measured?
    (1) Yogurt
    (2) Applesauce
    (3) Pureed peaches
    (4) Chocolate ice cream

20. A resident who is incontinent of feces says to the nurse, "This is disgusting. How can you stand this?" The nurse's *best* response would be:
    (1) "You sound upset?"
    (2) "This is disgusting?"
    (3) "I am used to this by now."
    (4) "It's not as bad as you think."

21. The Heimlich maneuver (abdominal thrust) attempts to:
    (1) Force air out of the lungs
    (2) Increase systemic circulation
    (3) Induce emptying of the stomach
    (4) Put pressure on the apex of the heart

22. Prior to discharge an aged patient complains that her feet always feel cold. To best keep her feet warm, the nurse should teach her to:
    (1) Wrap a blanket around them
    (2) Wear a pair of cotton socks
    (3) Submerge them in warm water
    (4) Place them on a heating pad

23. To clean an indwelling urinary catheter (Foley) when providing perineal care, the nurse should:
    (1) Scrub up and down the tube with soap and water
    (2) Wear a gown and gloves throughout the procedure
    (3) Wash a tubing before washing the urinary meatus
    (4) Bathe around the catheter moving away from the meatus

24. Growth and development progresses at a rate that can be described as:
    (1) Fast
    (2) Slow
    (3) Smooth
    (4) Irregular

25. When a fire is discovered in a dirty utility room, the nurse's FIRST action should be to:
    (1) Close the fire doors on the unit
    (2) Move patients toward the stairs
    (3) Attempt to put out the fire
    (4) Pull the fire alarm

26. When moving to a sitting position, the patient complains of dizziness. The initial response of the nurse should be to:
    (1) Position the patient's head between the knees
    (2) Transfer the patient to a bedside chair quickly
    (3) Instruct the patient to sit on the side of the bed
    (4) Tell the patient to stand at the bedside for a few minutes

27. Mrs. Benson is terminally ill. Which of the following is an unexpected behavior associated with the usual process of grieving?
    (1) Talking about the illness
    (2) Becoming angry with people

(3) Attempting to commit suicide
(4) Seeking alternative therapies

28. The patient has black tarry colored stools. The nurse recognizes that this is related to:
    (1) Overproduction of bile
    (2) Gastrointestinal bleeding
    (3) Decreased absorption of fat
    (4) Deficient pancreatic enzymes

29. When taking a patient's blood pressure, the nurse opens the pressure valve knob and the mercury drops quickly. The nurse should:
    (1) Remove the cuff and send the sygnomonometer for repair
    (2) Squeeze the air out of the cuff and try again
    (3) Wait 2 minutes before pumping up the cuff
    (4) Check the tubing and cuff for air leaks

30. Following surgery the most common reason patients will have a nasogastric tube in place is for the purpose of:
    (1) Decompression
    (2) Instillation
    (3) Lavage
    (4) Gavage

ANSWERS AND RATIONALES FOR PRACTICE TEST A

An asterisk (*) is in front of the rationale that explains the correct answer.

1. (1) This might send a message to the patient that could precipitate feelings of guilt or imply to the patient that the nurse no longer wanted to provide care.
  * (2) Anger is a defense or response to loss; the nurse must recognize that the patient is using displacement to deal with emotional pain.
    (3) This would abandon the patient at a time when the patient should be given an opportunity to verbalize feelings.
    (4) This is a defensive response that focuses on the nurse rather than the patient.

2. (1) This is unnecessary unless the patient had a concomitant neuromusculo-skeletal problem.
    (2) This is too long a period of time between the release of restaints and could result in contractures.
  * (3) Under usual circumstances, this is often enough to permit ROM exercises to prevent contractures.
    (4) Same as #2.

3. * (1) A patient's basic physical needs should be given first priority.
    (2) The patient should be cleaned first; the patient may not have the physical, mental, or emotional ability to achieve this goal.
    (3) Same as #2.
    (4) Same as #2.

4. * (1) Side rails provide a barrier that prevents the patient from falling out of bed; they also provide a hand-hold for turning or maintaining balance.
    (2) This is unsafe; this is a movable object that would not provide a stable barrier.
    (3) Repositioning could increase the risk of falling out of bed.
    (4) Although this decreases the sensation of being up high, it will not provide a barrier to prevent a fall.

5. (1) This is impractical; the patient cannot sit at the nurses' station all the time.
    (2) Patients should not be responsible for each other.
    (3) This is impractical; the nurse also must care for other patients.
  * (4) This reduces anxiety because the patient knows that someone will come immediately if help is needed.

6. (1) Fluids only given three times a day would not be adequate.
  * (2) The patient is dependent on the nurse because of the inability to be self-sufficient; frequent small amounts of fluid are more desirable than larger amounts of fluid less frequently.
    (3) This is useless because the patient is restrained.
    (4) This is unrealistic.

7. * (1) The weight of the chest and pressure of the abdominal organs against the diaphragm limit thoracic excursion causing dyspnea.
    (2) This position allows the abdominal organs to drop via gravity allowing the diaphragm to effectively contract promoting full expansion of the lungs.
    (3) Same as #2.
    (4) Same as #2.

8. (1) Although this would be documented, the patient's response to care is the most important fact.
    (2) Same as #1.
  * (3) This is most important because the patient's response will indicate if the care given was appropriate and effective and if future care should be altered.
    (4) Same as #1.

9. (1) Although this might be done later, listening comes first; open-ended questions are more therapeutic.
    (2) Although this might be done, listening comes first.
    (3) Same as #2.
  * (4) Reception of a message must occur before the nurse can intervene; by listening, the nurse collects information that will influence future care.

10. (1) This is an emotional-behavioral response to pain.
    (2) Same as #1.
  * (3) An increased heart rate is part of the fight-or-flight response, which is controlled by the autonomic nervous system; it is a physical attempt to prepare for an emergency.
    (4) Same as #1.

11. (1) Daily baths can remove protective oils and cause drying of the skin, which could compromise homeostasis.
  * (2) The use of soap and water with friction followed by rinsing the skin with water removes microorganisms on the skin.
    (3) Although soap reduces the surface tension of water, which facilitates cleaning, it is water and friction that primarily remove microorganisms and dirt from the skin.
    (4) These are not values held by all individuals.

12.   (1) Nursing assistants can refuse to perform tasks that are outside the parameters of their role and job responsibilities.
       (2) Health team members must have a professional relationship with mutual respect; they do not have to be friends.
       (3) Although the nursing assistant aide can be self-directed within the role, the nursing assistant must work under the direct supervision of a nurse.
     * (4) The responsibilities and job description of the nursing assistant must be clear to all members of the nursing team; nursing assistants should perform only those tasks that are within their role, have been learned, and have been assigned.

13.   (1) Decision making is difficult for patients who are cognitively impaired and confused.
       (2) Cognitively impaired patients may have difficulty comprehending the concepts of *good* and *all.*
     * (3) Simple direct statements are more easily understood by patients who are cognitively impaired and confused.
       (4) Cognitively impaired and confused patients have difficulty understanding the concept of *cause and effect.*

14.   (1) The lips still can form an effective seal around the thermometer to result in an accurate reading.
     * (2) Oxygen is cooling, and the resulting temperature would be abnormally low; some agencies permit oral temperatures when the patient has a nasal cannula.
       (3) An 8-year-old child is old enough to follow directions to safely obtain an accurate oral temperature.
       (4) Same as #1.

15.   (1) This is unsafe. The bag and tubing would be above the level of the patient's bladder; urine could flow backward into the bladder resulting in an urinary tract infection.
       (2) This is unsafe. The urinary collection bag would become contaminated; this is a violation of medical asepsis.
       (3) Same as #1.
     * (4) The urinary collection bag would be below the patient's bladder, and urine could flow by gravity; hanging it on the chair and keeping it off the floor supports medical asepsis.

16. * (1) Paralysis of the lower extremities results in reduced mobility; maintaining one position exposes the compressed capillary beds to pressure which causes tissue hypoxia resulting in decubitus ulcers.
       (2) A patient with hypotension is at risk for falls because hypotension can cause dizziness.
       (3) A patient with memory loss may have emotional or safety related problems.
       (4) A patient with heart failure is at risk for a dysrhythmia.

17. * (1) All patients in a hospital require care that employs medical aseptic techniques; procedures that break the chain of infection help control the transmission of microorganisms.
       (2) Not all patients require care that necessitates this specific intervention.
       (3) Same as #2.
       (4) Same as #2.

18.   (1) This is traumatic and could cause further bleeding.
       (2) This is unnecessary; the loss of a drop of blood would not influence vital signs.

* (3) Pressure constricts blood vessels which will limit bleeding; an antiseptic swab will help prevent infection at the needle insertion site.
  (4) This is unnecessary; although this is not an expected therapeutic response, it does occasionally occur because the needle may pierce a tiny blood vessel.

19.   (1) This is a solid.
     (2) Same as #1.
     (3) Same as #1.
  * (4) At room temperature ice cream melts, changing it from a solid to a liquid.

20. * (1) this is an example of reflective technique; it focuses on the patient's feelings and encourages verbalization.
     (2) Although this may encourage the patient to talk more, it focuses on the content of what the patient said rather than the emotional theme.
     (3) This denies the patient's feelings.
     (4) Same as #3.

21. * (1) The rise in intraabdominal and intrathoracic pressure and the abrupt jolt to the diaphragm uses air within the bronchial tree behind the obstruction to force out whatever is causing the obstruction in the trachea.
     (2) This occurs during cardiac compression associated with cardiopulmonary resuscitation (CPR).
     (3) The obstruction is in the trachea of the respiratory system, not the esophagus of the gastrointestinal system.
     (4) Same as #2.

22.   (1) This is unsafe; pressure on the toes and feet could produce footdrop.
  * (2) Socks trap body heat which keeps the feet warm; socks also absorb moisture and allow foot mobility.
     (3) This is impractical; this should be done to bathe the feet, not warm them. With decreased peripheral perception it could injure the tissues if the water was too warm.
     (4) This is unsafe; this could result in burns, particularly in the elderly who tend to have decreased peripheral perception.

23.   (1) This would move contaminated material toward the urinary meatus, which could result in an infection.
     (2) While gloves are appropriate for universal precautions, a gown is unnecessary.
     (3) Same as #1.
  * (4) This action supports the concept of cleansing from a clean area (urinary meatus) toward a dirty area (down the catheter and away from the meatus).

24.   (1) Growth and development are not continuously fast, although infants and adolescents experience growth spurts.
     (2) Growth and development are not continuously slow, although adults and the elderly may experience slower periods of growth.
     (3) Growth and development reflect change, and change is rarely smooth.
  * (4) Growth and development as a whole is uneven; some stages are faster than others and people move through the stages at their own pace. The commonalities of growth and development are predictable, but a specific individual's changes are unpredictable.

25.   (1) This may eventually be done, but it is not the priority.
     (2) Same as #1.

   (3) Same as #1.
 * (4) Of the options presented, this would be the nurse's first action; this alerts other health team members and the fire department that help is needed.

26. (1) This is unsafe; it moves the patient's center of gravity forward, and the patient could fall.
     (2) This is unsafe; this would not permit time for the patient's vasomotor response to compensate for the change in position, and the patient could fall.
   * (3) Orthostatic or postural hypotension occurs because the ability of the autonomic nervous system to equalize the blood supply is diminished with bed rest. When rising, blood pools in the lower extremities until the sympathetic nervous system causes peripheral vasoconstriction; sitting on the side of the bed for a few minutes gives the body time to adjust.
     (4) Same as #2.

27. (1) Although this behavior occurs throughout the grieving response, it is most expected during the early stage of denial and disbelief ("No, not me").
     (2) Anger is expected and occurs when there is a developing awareness of the impending loss ("Yes me").
   * (3) Although some people who are terminally ill attempt suicide, it is not a normal expected response to loss.
     (4) This behavior occurs most often during the stage of bargaining ("Yes me, but").

28. (1) Bile pigments color the stool brown; in the absence of bile pigments, stool has a clay color.
   * (2) Digestive acids and enzymes act on blood in the gastrointestinal system causing the stool to become back or tarry in color.
     (3) In the absence of pancreatic enzymes there is a decreased absorption of fat resulting in stool that contains white globules of fat and is foul smelling.
     (4) Same as #3.

29. (1) This should be unnecessary; before being applied to the patient's arm, the sygnomonometer should have been checked for proper functioning.
     (2) This is unsafe; pumping the cuff too soon traps excess blood in the extremity resulting in an inaccurate reading and possible discomfort.
   * (3) This allows for venous return and prevents falsely elevated results.
     (4) Same as #1.

30. * (1) Negative pressure exerted through a tube inserted in the stomach removes secretions and gaseous substances from the stomach, preventing abdominal distention.
     (2) This is not the most common purpose of a nasogastric tube following surgery; instillations in a nasogastric tube following surgery are done to promote patency.
     (3) This is not the most common purpose of a nasogastric tube following surgery; lavage following surgery is usually done to promote hemostasis in the presence of gastric bleeding.
     (4) This would be contraindicated following surgery until peristalsis returns.

PRACTICE TEST B

1. The patient had a stroke (cerebral vascular accident) and is paralyzed on the right side (hemiplegia). When undressing the patient, the nurse should:

(1) Take the gown off the right side first
(2) Get assistance when undressing the patient
(3) Remove the gown from the left side before the right
(4) Sit the patient up to make undressing less stressful

2. To foster a patient's self-esteem needs, the nurse's best intervention would be to:
(1) Place an identification band on the patient's wrist
(2) Answer the patient's call light immediately
(3) Compliment the patient on his appearance
(4) Encourage the patient to make choices

3. When a patient is having a seizure while out of bed, the nurse's initial action should be to:
(1) Move the patient back to bed
(2) Get an airway and portable oxygen
(3) Move objects away from around the patient
(4) Hold the patient's arms and legs securely

4. To best promote healthy teeth, the nurse should teach patients to:
(1) Drink milk daily
(2) Eat a high-calcium diet
(3) Brush the teeth after eating
(4) Visit the dentist every year

5. The factor that *most* upsets adults who are incontinent is the feeling of:
(1) Dependence
(2) Regression
(3) Loneliness
(4) Wetness

6. Mr. Weinstein is at risk for dehydration and has "Force Fluids" ordered by the physician. To increase Mr. Weinstein's intake of fluid, the nurse should:
(1) Measure all fluid intake and urine output
(2) Explain that a feeding tube may have to be used
(3) Require him to drink 4 ounces of fluid every hour
(4) Provide drinks he likes and assist him in drinking

7. The nurse needs to recognize that the patient MOST likely to become constipated would be a patient who:
(1) Leads a sedentary lifestyle
(2) Is on a low-sodium diet
(3) Works sitting at a desk
(4) Eats pears and peas

8. One factor common to all communication is the:
(1) Direction of the message
(2) Fact that there is a message
(3) Transmission route
(4) Use of words

9. Which of the following should be assessed further?
(1) A pulse rate that is 68 and regular
(2) A respiratory rate of 28 per minute
(3) A blood pressure reading of 120/88
(4) A rectal temperature of 99.8°F

10. When people are on complete bed rest, their hair tends to become:
(1) Oily
(2) Dry

(3) Sparse
(4) Matted

11. A patient is disoriented to time and place and has impaired cognitive ability because of extensive brain damage following a motor vehicle accident. When administering care, the nurse should:
    (1) Offer basic choices
    (2) Explain care in detail
    (3) Provide simple directions
    (4) Teach activities of daily living

12. When measuring an elderly patient's height, the patient says, "I am now 1 inch shorter than I was as a young woman." The nurse should:
    (1) Explain that people do not usually lose height
    (2) Recognize this as part of growth and development
    (3) Understand that this could be the sign of a problem
    (4) Identify that the patient is worried about her height

13. When a patient does not sleep well at night, the most effective nursing intervention would be to:
    (1) Encourage the patient to avoid daytime naps
    (2) Fix the patient a warm cup of tea before bedtime
    (3) Tell the patient to take a long walk before bedtime
    (4) Obtain a physician's order for a sleeping medication

14. A patient with a terminal illness says to the nurse, "Do you believe in life after death?" The nurse's most therapeutic response would be:
    (1) "I don't know."
    (2) "What do you think?"
    (3) "Why are you asking?"
    (4) "That's a difficult question."

15. Mr. Glass is immobile and is on a turning and positioning schedule. When turning Mr. Glass, the nurse identifies a small red area on the coccyx. The nurse's initial intervention should be to:
    (1) Apply a warm soak to the area
    (2) Expose the area to a heat lamp
    (3) Order an air mattress for the bed
    (4) Massage around the area with skin lotion

16. Mr. Koch has a small infected decubitus ulcer and is on drainage-secretion isolation. When providing a bed bath, what should the nurse wear in addition to gloves?
    (1) A face mask
    (2) A clean gown
    (3) A disposable hat
    (4) A pair of eye glasses

17. A semi-Fowler's position is used to:
    (1) Reduce development of decubitus ulcers
    (2) Minimize flexion contractures of the hip
    (3) Relieve pressure on ischial tuberosities
    (4) Prevent aspiration during nasogastric tube feeding

18. The major difference between acute and chronic pain is that chronic pain is usually:
    (1) Severe
    (2) Relentless
    (3) Unbearable
    (4) Predictable

19. The patient is on a therapeutic diet that includes liquid supplements. The nurse should serve the supplements:
    (1) Between meals
    (2) When they arrive on the unit
    (3) Whenever the patient is hungry
    (4) If the patient eats less than 50 percent of a meal

20. Mrs. Hallow has a below-the-knee amputation. She explains to the nurse that she would rather put on her prosthesis while sitting in a chair. The nurse should:
    (1) Compromise and attach the leg while the patient sits on the bed
    (2) Teach her to put the prosthesis on while lying in bed
    (3) Explain that it is unsafe to transfer with one leg
    (4) Write this preference on the nursing care plan

21. To effectively put out a fire, the nurse should direct the spray from the fire extinguisher across the:
    (1) Middle of the flames
    (2) Edge of the flames
    (3) Base of the flames
    (4) Top of the flames

22. Mrs. Kay has a full body cast and is experiencing diarrhea. She is at high risk for developing:
    (1) Decubitus ulcers
    (2) A wound infection
    (3) Urinary incontinence
    (4) A hip flexion contracture

23. A patient's vital signs are oral temperature 99°F, pulse 84 with a regular rhythm, respirations 16 and deep, and blood pressure 180/110. The sign that should cause the most concern for the nurse would be the:
    (1) Pulse
    (2) Temperature
    (3) Respirations
    (4) Blood pressure

24. When providing perineal care to a female patient, the nurse should NEVER:
    (1) Wash the vaginal area before the buttocks
    (2) Let the patient bathe herself
    (3) Rub the area dry
    (4) Use soap

25. When inserting a vaginal cream, the nurse's initial action should be to:
    (1) Apply a lubricant to the applicator
    (2) Put on sterile gloves for the procedure
    (3) Perform perineal care with soap and water
    (4) Place the patient in the left-side-lying position

26. Mr. Stein has been told by his physician that he has metastatic lung cancer and he is seriously ill. After a severe episode of coughing and shortness of breath, he says to the nurse, "This is just a cold. I'll be fine once I get over it." The nurse's best response would be:
    (1) "Remember what the doctor told you this morning."
    (2) "The doctor had some bad news for you today."
    (3) "It's not a cold, it's lung cancer."
    (4) "Tell me more about your illness."

27. When transferring a patient who is weak on the right side from the bed to a chair, the nurse should:
    (1) Place the feet of the patient close together
    (2) Plan to use a mechanical lift for the transfer
    (3) Instruct the patient to bear weight equally on both legs
    (4) Put the right arm of the chair against the left side of the bed

28. Which of the following signs is unrelated to hypoxia?
    (1) Jaundice
    (2) Cyanosis
    (3) Pallor
    (4) Dusky

29. When administering an enema, the patient complains of abdominal cramping. The nurse should:
    (1) Lower the fluid container several inches
    (2) Stop the fluid until the cramping subsides
    (3) Turn the patient to the right lateral position
    (4) Have the patient flex the knees toward the abdomen

30. When assessing a patient's respiratory status during recovery from anesthesia, it is of primary importance for the nurse to evaluate the patient's ability to:
    (1) Inhale voluntarily
    (2) Breathe deeply
    (3) Swallow
    (4) Speak

ANSWERS AND RATIONALES FOR PRACTICE TEST B

An asterisk (*) is in front of the rationale that explains the correct answer.

1.   (1) This is unsafe; this exerts excessive stress on the affected side.
    (2) The patient needs assistance with undressing, and this activity can be safely performed by one nurse.
    * (3) This exerts less stress on the affected side; the unaffected side can better tolerate the tension or positioning required to remove the gown.
    (4) This is irrelevant; the gown should be removed from the left side first whether the patient is standing, sitting, or lying down.

2.   (1) This meets needs associated with safety and security.
    (2) Same as #1.
    (3) This provides external, rather than internal, reinforcement of self-esteem.
    * (4) This promotes self-control, dignity, and individuality, which all support self-esteem; it provides independence which is a form of internal reinforcement of worth. Internal reinforcement of worth is usually more beneficial than external reinforcement.

3.   (1) This is unsafe; restriction of movement or manipulation of limbs during the tonic-clonic phase of a seizure could result in fractures or tissue damage.
    (2) Physical safety is the priority at this time; the patient will not breathe until the convulsive phase of the seizure is over at which time this may be done.
    * (3) Physical safety is the priority; the patient's uncontrolled movements could result in injury if environmental obstacles are not removed from the patient's immediate vicinity.
    (4) Same as #1.

4.   (1) Although this provides calcium, it will not prevent dental caries or gingivitis.
     (2) Same as #1.
   * (3) Friction removes food particles and other debris that cause dental caries and gingivitis.
     (4) Although helpful, dentists usually limit problems rather than prevent them; oral hygiene several times daily, including brushing and flossing, is the best measure for promoting healthy teeth.

5.   (1) Not all people who are incontinent are dependent on others; many people are capable of cleaning themselves.
   * (2) Incontinence is often associated with childlike behavior; most cultures value control over one's bodily functions, which is usually accomplished early in life.
     (3) Although incontinence is embarrassing, which may result in social isolation and loneliness, it is the feeling of being like a child that causes the most concern.
     (4) Although being wet and soiled are uncomfortable, it is the feelings associated with regression that are most upsetting.

6.   (1) This will document the patient's intake and output, but it will do nothing to promote intake.
     (2) This is a threat, and the nurse could be held accountable for assault.
     (3) This is a form of force and is unacceptable; the patient has a right to refuse. The patient should be taught the importance of fluid intake.
   * (4) Providing for patient preferences increases the likelihood of the patient accepting the fluid; encouragement and support are motivating, which may increase fluid intake.

7. * (1) People who are inactive have decreased peristalsis which increases water reabsorption in the large intestine promoting constipation.
     (2) This is unrelated to constipation.
     (3) Although this could reduce peristalsis, it does not address the patient's entire lifestyle; a patient with a job that does not require physical activity can exercise at other times.
     (4) These contain fiber which increases intestinal peristalsis promoting defecation.

8.   (1) Messages go in a variety of directions (e.g., from the nurse to the patient, from the patient to the nurse).
   * (2) Communication is the transfer of information from one person to another; in communication there is always a message.
     (3) A message can be transmitted via a variety of routes (e.g., verbal, nonverbal).
     (4) Communication can be nonverbal (e.g., touch, a smile).

9.   (1) This is within the normal range of 60 to 80 beats per minute and the rhythm is regular, indicating no abnormalities.
   * (2) This is above the normal range of 14 to 20 breaths per minute and is abnormal.
     (3) This is within the normal range of 100 to 140 mm Hg for the systolic reading and 60 to 90 mm Hg for the diastolic reading, indicating no abnormalities.
     (4) This is within the normal range of 97.6 to 99.8°F for a rectal temperature, indicating no abnormalities.

10. (1) This is caused by lack of washing the hair, not bed rest.
     (2) This is caused by nutrition and endocrine problems, not bed rest; brushing will help disperse natural secretions down the shaft of the hair.

(3) This is caused by nutrition, endocrine, and genetic factors, not bed rest.

* (4) Pressure and friction of the hair against the pillow results in matted, tangled hair.

11. (1) This is too challenging a task for a person with extensive brain damage.

(2) Patients with extensive brain damage lack the cognitive ability to integrate details or comprehend *cause and effect.*

* (3) Simple, short statements with a single message are the easiest to intellectually integrate.

(4) Same as #1.

12. (1) This is untrue; people do get shorter as they age.

* (2) Compression of the vertebral column causes people to get slightly shorter as they age.

(3) This is untrue; losing height is an expected response to aging.

(4) Nothing in the patient's statement indicates anxiety; it is a declarative statement.

13. * (1) Naps rest and restore the body, reducing the need to sleep longer at night; an active routine throughout the day requires energy that promotes a need for sleep at night.

(2) This is contraindicated; tea contains caffeine which is a stimulant that will interfere with the ability to fall asleep.

(3) This increases the basal metabolic rate, which would interfere with sleep if done immediately before bedtime; exercise should be performed earlier in the day.

(4) Other measures such as avoiding daytime naps, exercising during the day, drinking milk (which contains L-Tryptophan), and performing usual bedtime routines should be attempted before medication.

14. (1) Although this is a direct response to the patient's question, it does not focus on the patient's concerns.

* (2) This focuses on the patient's concern and provides an opportunity to verbalize further.

(3) This is too confrontational and may cut off communication.

(4) This side-steps the patient's question and may or may not promote further dialogue.

15. (1) This requires a physician's order.

(2) Same as #1.

(3) This may be done later; while the area is exposed, the nurse should massage around the area with lotion to promote circulation.

* (4) Friction increases blood, oxygen, and nutrients to the area which promote healing.

16. (1) This is unnecessary; this is used for respiratory isolation where microorganisms are transmitted by respiratory droplets.

* (2) A gown protects the nurse's uniform from contact with contaminated material; it acts as a barrier and interrupts the chain of infection.

(3) This is used for strict isolation.

(4) This is unnecessary in this situation; a protective eye shield may be used for a large wound with extensive drainage where spattering is likely to occur.

17.   (1) This position increases pressure over the sacrum, posterior iliac crests, and ischial tuberosities.
       (2) This position can cause hip flexion contractures if the patient's position is unchanged for prolonged periods of time.
       (3) Same as #1.
     * (4) Raising the head of the bed keeps the nasogastric tube feeding in the stomach via the principle of gravity.

18.   (1) Both acute and chronic pain can have this characteristic.
     * (2) Chronic pain lasts over a prolonged period of time; acute pain usually has a short duration.
       (3) Same as #1.
       (4) Same as #1.

19. * (1) Supplements imply *in addition to* and therefore should be supplied between meals.
       (2) They should be offered between meals or when specifically ordered; supplements may be sent to the unit long before the time they should be offered, particularly if they are canned commercial formulas.
       (3) This could interfere with the intake of the patient's ordered meals.
       (4) The patient should be encouraged to eat the entire meal; formulas should supplement, not substitute, the diet.

20.   (1) This negates the patient's right to individualized care.
       (2) Same as #1.
       (3) This is untrue; if all the principles of body mechanics are followed, a safe transfer can be performed on one leg.
     * (4) The patient has the right to individualized care; communicating patient preferences on the nursing care plan promotes continuity of care.

21.   (1) This is unsafe; this could scatter the burning debris which would intensify the fire.
       (2) Same as #1.
     * (3) The source of the fire is at its base where the fuel (e.g., linens, paper, inflammable liquids) is burning.
       (4) This is ineffective; this is too far from the source of the burning material.

22. * (1) In addition to being warm and moist, feces contain enzymes that promote tissue breakdown.
       (2) There is no wound present to become infected; fecal material could cause a vaginal or urinary tract infection, not a wound infection.
       (3) Immobility may precipitate urinary retention rather than incontinence; diarrhea would not promote urinary incontinence.
       (4) With a full body cast the hips are usually in extension.

23.   (1) Although this is slightly outside the normal range of 70 to 80 beats per minute, the rhythm is regular; the nurse should assess the patient further and compare it to this patient's baseline data.
       (2) This is within the normal range of 97.6 to 99.6°F for an oral temperature
       (3) This is within the normal range of 14 to 20 breaths per minute.
     * (4) The blood pressure is above the normal range of 100 to 140 mm Hg for the systolic reading and 60 to 90 mm Hg for the diastolic reading and should cause the most concern of the options presented.

24. (1) This supports the principle of washing from clean to dirty which is an acceptable practice; it cleanses microorganisms away from the urinary meatus and vagina.

(2) This would support the patient's privacy and promote dignity and independence.

* (3) This is unsafe; rubbing could damage the delicate perineal tissue; the area should be patted dry.

(4) Soap lowers the surface tension of water, which promotes cleaning of the perineal area.

25. (1) This is unnecessary; a portion of the vaginal cream is ejected at the tip of the applicator just prior to and during insertion, which lubricates the applicator.

(2) This is unnecessary; this is not a sterile procedure. Clean gloves are adequate.

* (3) Vaginal creams are usually administered to treat vaginal infections or discharges; the area must be bathed to remove secretions and microorganisms immediately prior to the administration of medication.

(4) The dorsal recumbent position is used for vaginal insertions.

26. (1) This would take away the patient's coping mechanism, is demeaning, and could cut off communication; the patient is using denial to cope with the diagnosis.

(2) Same as #1.

(3) Same as #1.

* (4) This provides an opportunity to discuss the illness; eventually a developing awareness will occur, and the patient will move on to other coping mechanisms.

27. (1) This eliminates a wide base of support and raises the center of gravity which promotes falls.

(2) This is unnecessary; a patient with hemiparesis is capable of transferring with assistance. A mechanical lift promotes dependency and eliminates an opportunity to strengthen the unaffected leg.

(3) This is unrealistic and unsafe; the side with the hemiparesis cannot bear as much weight as the unaffected side.

* (4) The patient with a hemiparesis should get out of bed by leading with the unaffected side; this allows the stronger arm and leg to lead the movement into a chair. A patient with a right hemiparesis should get out of the left side of the bed.

28. * (1) This is a yellow-orange discoloration of the skin, mucous membrane, and sclera caused by elevated blood levels of bilirubin, which deposits bile pigments into tissues.

(2) This is a blue discoloration of the skin and mucous membranes caused by deoxygenated hemoglobin in the capillaries; it is a late sign of hypoxia.

(3) This is an unnatural paleness or decreased color in the skin caused by reduced amounts of oxyhemoglobin.

(4) This is a grayish discoloration of the skin, which frequently indicates deoxygenated hemoglobin in the capillaries in people with dark skin.

29. (1) This would still allow fluid to enter the colon, continuing the problem of abdominal cramping.

* (2) This interrupts the flow of fluid which is distending and irritating the bowel; it reduces intestinal pressure and allows the intestinal cramping to subside.

(3) This raises intraabdominal pressure, which may precipitate evacuation of the enema fluid from the bowel.

(4) Same as #3.

30. (1) Although a patient may still be unconscious, the patient usually breathes spontaneously; the respiratory center in the brain stem is responsible for the involuntary control of breathing.

(2) After the patient recovers from anesthesia, then coughing and deep breathing become important to prevent atelectasis and pneumonia.

* (3) Anesthesia interferes with the gag reflex; until the gag reflex returns, the patient cannot safely swallow without a risk of aspiration.

(4) This is unrelated to the patient's respiratory status.

PRACTICE TEST C

1. To help prevent injury to a patient with bone demineralization, the nurse should:
   (1) Apply emollients to the skin every day
   (2) Have the patient walk in the hall once daily
   (3) Support the patient's joints when turning and moving
   (4) Encourage the patient to drink 2500 ml of fluid daily

2. The nurse should brush a patient's hair daily to prevent:
   (1) Pediculosis
   (2) Dandruff
   (3) Alopecia
   (4) Tangles

3. A patient has a progressive, debilitating disease. Although he is usually pleasant, he begins to complain that the doctor is incompetent, the nurses are uncaring, the room is too cold, and the food is terrible. The patient is coping by using the defense mechanism of:
   (1) Displacement
   (2) Projection
   (3) Denial
   (4) Anger

4. When an assessment reveals a change in a patient's blood pressure, the nurse should first:
   (1) Report the change to the charge nurse
   (2) Document the observed change
   (3) Obtain the other vital signs
   (4) Notify the physician

5. Which of the following actions by a patient should be reported to the physician because the patient may need a restraint?
   (1) Climbing off the end of the bed at night
   (2) Wandering into other patients' rooms
   (3) Picking at the gown and bed linens
   (4) Falling asleep when in a chair

6. A comatose patient begins to vomit while lying in bed. The nurse's initial response should be to position the patient in the:
   (1) Supine position
   (2) Lateral position
   (3) Fowler's position
   (4) Dorsal recumbent position

7. Mrs. Timmons, whose husband recently died, begins to cry. The nurse's best response would be to:
   (1) Look away when she cries
   (2) Sit down and touch her hand
   (3) Arrange for grief counseling
   (4) Explain that being sad is normal

8. The nurse would recognize that Mr. Alverez received an adequate night's sleep when he:
   (1) Demonstrates renewed strength
   (2) Sleeps at night without waking
   (3) Is able to remember his dreams
   (4) Slept a minimum of 7 hours

9. Ethics is specifically concerned with:
   (1) Preventing a crime
   (2) Protecting civil law
   (3) Determining right or wrong
   (4) Potentially negligent actions

10. When feeding a patient with left-sided hemiparesis due to a stroke, the nurse should:
    (1) Position the patient in a low-Fowler's position
    (2) Offer fluids to assist with swallowing food
    (3) Place food on the strong side of the mouth
    (4) Position a towel under the patient's chin

11. Mr. Valente has a left-sided hemiplegia as the result of a cerebral vascular accident. While assisting him to dress, he states in a disgusted tone of voice, "I feel like a 2-year-old. I can't even get dressed by myself." The nurse's BEST response would be:
    (1) "It must be hard to feel dependent on others."
    (2) "Most people who have had a stroke feel this way."
    (3) "It must be horrible not being able to move your arm."
    (4) "You are feeling down today, but things will get better."

12. A newly admitted patient complains of not having had a good bowel movement in 10 days. Which of the following questions asked by the nurse would identify symptoms of a fecal impaction?
    (1) "What types of food with fiber do you eat?"
    (2) "Do you notice a bad odor to your breath?"
    (3) "Have you had small amounts of liquid stool?"
    (4) "Are you experiencing any nausea and vomiting?"

13. Mrs. Vane is on isolation. The <u>most</u> effective way to reduce the transmission of microorganisms at mealtime is by:
    (1) Using disposable dishes and utensils
    (2) Washing and rinsing the dishes with hot water
    (3) Having the patient wash her hands after eating
    (4) Isolating her used tray in the dirty utility room

14. Which of the following actions utilizes poor body mechanics?
    (1) Flexing the knees when lifting an object from the floor
    (2) Holding clean equipment close to the body when walking
    (3) Placing the feet apart when transferring a patient
    (4) Bending from the waist when making a bed

15. A dying patient says to the nurse, "I was much more religious when I was young." The nurse's *best* response would be:
    (1) "Do you still believe in God?"
    (2) "Do you want us to pray for you?"

(3) "Would you like me to call a chaplain?"
(4) "Are you concerned about life after death?"

16. When giving a complete bed bath, of the following, what body part should the nurse wash last?
    (1) Legs
    (2) Feet
    (3) Rectum
    (4) Axilla

17. A patient has a sacral decubitus ulcer. To reduce pressure to the sacral area, the nurse should position the patient in the:
    (1) Dorsal recumbent position
    (2) Semi-Fowler's position
    (3) Lateral position
    (4) Supine position

18. When instilling ear drops into the ear of a young child, the nurse should:
    (1) Hyperextend the head prior to instilling the drops
    (2) Apply pressure to the tragus of the ear while instilling the drops
    (3) Pull the pinna of the ear downward and backward while instilling the drops
    (4) Maintain the side-lying position with the affected ear down after instilling the drops

19. The bed of a patient with an indwelling urinary catheter (Foley) is always wet with urine. The nurse should:
    (1) Insert a larger-size catheter
    (2) Provide perineal care whenever necessary
    (3) Position a waterproof pad under the patient's buttocks
    (4) Tell the patient to use the bedpan when needing to void

20. The location and characteristics of pain are important for the nurse to explore when determining its:
    (1) Etiology
    (2) Duration
    (3) Threshold
    (4) Intensity

21. A Class A fire extinguisher can put out a fire in a:
    (1) Toaster oven
    (2) Maintenance closest
    (3) Wastepaper basket
    (4) Stove in the pantry

22. When providing mouth care for the unconscious patient, the nurse should:
    (1) Explain to the patient what will be done and why
    (2) Apply KY jelly (lubricant) to the tongue and lips
    (3) Use glycerine and lemon swabs to cleanse the mouth
    (4) Position the patient in the dorsal recumbent position

23. Across the spectrum of wellness and illness, *most* elderly people view themselves as:
    (1) Tired
    (2) Healthy
    (3) Infirmed
    (4) Dependent

24. Mrs. Jones is intermittently disoriented to time and place and is unsteady when ambulating. When assisting her to meet elimination needs, the nurse should:
    (1) Have her use the bedpan while in bed
    (2) Encourage her to use a bedside commode

(3) Stay at her side while she is on the toilet
(4) Observe her through a slightly opened bathroom door

25. A patient with kidney failure is placed on fluid restrictions of 1000 ml of fluid in 24 hours. The nurse should:
    (1) Eliminate liquids between mealtimes
    (2) Divide the fluids equally among the three shifts
    (3) Indicate just clear liquids in the restriction plan
    (4) Proportion more fluids in the day than during the night

26. Which of the following patient assessments made by the nurse would require immediate intervention?
    (1) Rattling sounds in the pharynx of an unconscious patient
    (2) Coughing and expectorating large amounts of thick mucus
    (3) Moderate shortness of breath after returning from the bathroom
    (4) 10 respirations per minute by a sleeping patient

27. Which of the following actions by the nurse would support a patient's right to privacy?
    (1) Leaving a crying patient alone
    (2) Addressing a patient by the last name
    (3) Providing information about patient care
    (4) Pulling a curtain when interviewing the patient

28. When obtaining an oral temperature with an electronic thermometer, the nurse must:
    (1) Use the red probe
    (2) Take the temperature before breakfast
    (3) Use a new probe cover for each patient
    (4) Wipe the probe with alcohol after each use

29. When washing the penis of an uncircumcised patient, the nurse should:
    (1) Wash down the shaft toward the meatus
    (2) Retract the foreskin completely
    (3) Employ a very light touch
    (4) Use a rubbing motion

30. To prevent pulmonary complications postoperatively, the patient should be instructed to perform:
    (1) Incisional splinting
    (2) Progressive ambulation
    (3) Diaphragmatic breathing
    (4) Range-of-motion exercises

ANSWERS AND RATIONALES FOR PRACTICE TEST C

An asterisk (*) is in front of the rationale that explains the correct answer.

1.   (1) Emollients hold moisture in the skin making it supple; they do not prevent bone injury.
      (2) Weight bearing helps limit bone demineralization, but it will not prevent bone injury.
    * (3) Bone demineralization (osteoporosis) causes the bones to become weak, brittle, and fragile; supporting joints when turning or moving limits stress that could cause a fracture.
      (4) This flushes the kidneys and limits calculi formation which can occur because of the high level of calcium salts in the urine; however, it does not prevent bone injury.

2.   (1) Pediculosis is caused by direct contact with lice or their eggs (nits); brushing the hair will not prevent head lice.
      (2) Shampooing the hair and rubbing the scalp helps to limit dandruff.
      (3) Loss of hair is caused by nutritional, emotional, iatrogenic, and genetic factors; it is not prevented by brushing.
    * (4) Brushing separates tangles and evenly distributes secretions and oils down the hair shafts.

3. * (1) The patient is angry and is reducing the anxiety by transferring emotions from something stressful to substitutes, which are less anxiety producing.
      (2) This is the attribution of unacceptable thoughts or actions to another.
      (3) This is a defense mechanism with which the patient avoids emotional conflicts by refusing to consciously acknowledge thoughts or feelings.
      (4) Anger is a behavior that is an adaptive response; it defends the individual, but is not known as a defense mechanism.

4.   (1) This may be done after the other vital signs are obtained; corroborative data should be collected.
      (2) Same as #1.
    * (3) Because of the interrelationships among the circulatory system, respiratory system, and the basal metabolic rate, all the vital signs should be obtained for a significant assessment.
      (4) Same as #1.

5. * (1) This could result in self-harm, a factor indicating the need for a restraint.
      (2) This should be controlled by observation, not a restraint.
      (3) This is not unsafe behavior that requires application of a restraint.
      (4) This should be controlled by individualizing the patient's care with appropriate rest periods.

6.   (1) This is contraindicated; this promotes aspiration because it allows vomitus to flow to the posterior oral pharynx and enter the trachea.
    * (2) This prevents aspiration because it allows vomitus to drain out of the mouth via gravity.
      (3) This position would be inappropriate for an unconscious patient.
      (4) Same as #1.

7.   (1) This may give the patient the message that it is not acceptable to cry.
    * (2) This communicates acceptance and caring.

    (3) Although this may be done later, the patient needs immediate support.

    (4) Although this statement is often true, the nurse is making an assumption that the patient is sad; not knowing the patient-spouse relationship, the tears may indicate other feelings such as relief or joy.

8. * (1) The purpose of sleep is to rest and restore the body, which would be evidenced by renewed strength.

    (2) Although a person sleeps at night without waking, the length of the sleep or the length of REM sleep may be insufficient to restore or renew the body.

    (3) This is unrelated to adequate sleep; actually most dreams occur during REM sleep and are forgotten.

    (4) Seven hours may or may not be enough sleep because each person has unique needs and a biological clock for determining sleeping intervals.

9.   (1) Criminal law is concerned with crimes.

    (2) Civil law is concerned with wrongs committed by one person against another.

 * (3) Ethics is concerned with value judgments such as right and wrong or behavior that is acceptable or unacceptable.

    (4) Negligence is concerned with a careless act of commission or omission that results in injury to another.

10. (1) This could promote aspiration; the patient should be placed in a high-Fowler's position to allow gravity to facilitate swallowing.

    (2) This is contraindicated; this would promote aspiration; fluids should be taken after a mouthful of food is swallowed.

 * (3) This allows the unaffected muscles to control chewing, move the bolus of food to the posterior oral cavity, and facilitate swallowing.

    (4) This should be avoided because it has the same implication as a bib; the patient may feel childlike.

11. * (1) This identifies the patient's feelings and provides an opportunity for further discussion.

    (2) This is a generalization that may not be true; it also cuts off communication.

    (3) This focuses on the inability to move, rather than feelings of helplessness, dependence, and regression.

    (4) This is false reassurance because the nurse does not know if things will get better.

12. (1) This is not significant at this time; foods with fiber promote intestinal peristalsis which prevents constipation.

    (2) This is unrelated to fecal impaction; it may be related to a small bowel obstruction.

 * (3) A fecal impaction is an obstruction in the large intestine; peristalsis behind the obstruction initially increases in an attempt to move the mass, causing liquid stool to pass around the area of the impaction.

    (4) People with a fecal impaction may experience rectal pressure, bloating, and nausea, but rarely do they vomit; nausea and vomiting occur more frequently with small bowel obstructions.

13. * (1) Contaminated disposable articles can be double-bagged to contain microorganisms, which prevents their spread to others.

    (2) This is ineffective; boiling for 15 minutes will achieve disinfection.

(3) The hands should be washed before eating.

(4) This would contaminate the dirty utility room.

14.   (1) This is desirable because the strong muscles of the legs carry the load which helps prevent back strain.

(2) This is desirable because the weight is being carried close to the center of gravity, which helps maintain balance.

(3) The wider the base of support and the lower the center of gravity, the greater the stability of the nurse.

* (4) This puts too much stress on the vertebrae and muscles of the back because it does not distribute the work among the largest and strongest muscle groups of the legs.

15.   (1) This is inappropriate probing and would violate the patient's right to privacy or may put the patient on the defensive.

(2) This is an inappropriate question; not all the nurses on the team may want to assume this intervention.

* (3) This recognizes that the patient is considering personal spiritual needs; it provides an opportunity that the patient can accept or reject.

(4) Same as #1.

16.   (1) This area is cleaner than the perianal area, and if washed last, would become more contaminated from microorganisms and fecal material from the rectum.

(2) Same as #1.

* (3) The perianal area has fecal material and microorganisms that would contaminate other parts of the body; therefore, the perianal area should be washed last.

(4) Same as #1.

17.   (1) Pressure would still be on the sacrum because it is a back-lying position.

(2) Pressure would still be on the sacrum, and with the head elevated, shearing force could occur if the patient slides down in bed.

* (3) In this position the iliac crests and greater trochanter bear the body's weight.

(4) Same as #1.

18.   (1) This is done for the instillation of nose drops, not ear drops.

(2) This would prevent the drops from entering the ear canal.

* (3) This is done to straighten the ear canal in a child, which provides direct access to the deeper external ear structures; adults would have the ear pulled back and upward since the canal is straighter in the adult.

(4) This is contraindicated; this would allow the ear drops to flow out of the ear by gravity. The affected ear should be on the upper side for a minimum of 3 minutes to allow for complete distribution of the medication.

19.   * (1) Urine is leaking around the Foley catheter and a larger-size catheter is required; once the physician orders a Foley catheter, it is within the role of the nurse to select the appropriate size and perform the catheter insertion.

(2) With a Foley catheter in place, the patient should not be wet with urine because it is a closed system from the bladder to the collection bag; perineal care is performed routinely.

(3) This should be unnecessary because with an adequate-size catheter there should be no leaking of urine.

(4) The presence of a Foley catheter negates the need to void.

20. * (1) The location of pain is often related to the underlying disease or illness. The quality or subjective characteristics of pain often have common descriptions related to specific illness, such as burning pain associated with gastric ulcers and crushing chest pain associated with myocardial infarctions.
    (2) The length of time of the pain is not as significant as its location and characteristics in determining its etiology.
    (3) This is totally individual and unreliable for determining relationships among characteristics, location, or etiology of pain.
    (4) Same as #3.

21.   (1) A Class A fire extinguisher is contraindicated in an electrical fire because water conducts electricity.
    (2) A maintenance closet usually contains flammable materials; water is contraindicated because it dilutes flammable liquids, which spreads the fire.
  * (3) A Class A fire extinguisher contains water which safely and effectively puts out fires consisting of wood, paper, or cloth.
    (4) Water should not be used because it causes grease to spatter; also the stove might be an electric stove.

22. * (1) Hearing is the last sense to deteriorate, and the patient may hear the nurse; all patients have a right to know what will be done and why.
    (2) KY jelly is for external use.
    (3) These swabs should be applied after the mouth is cleansed.
    (4) This is contraindicated; this position would promote aspiration.

23.   (1) Although people lead more sedentary lifestyles as they age, they are still active; most elderly people do not view themselves as tired.
  * (2) Studies demonstrate that most elderly people perceive themselves as healthy because they measure their health in relation to how well they function rather than by the absence or presence of disease.
    (3) This is untrue; the majority of elderly are or perceive themselves as being independent, healthy, and active even if they have several chronic illnesses.
    (4) Same as #3.

24.   (1) This is unnecessary; the patient safely can go to the bathroom with assistance; a normal routine and position should be encouraged.
    (2) Same as #1.
  * (3) The patient needs supervision and assistance to prevent falls while maintaining as normal a routine as possible.
    (4) This is unsafe; the patient could fall without direct supervision.

25.   (1) Liquid intake should be dispersed over the hours when the patient is awake and not just ingested with meals.
    (2) This is inappropriate; patients should have more fluids during the day and evening than at night when they are usually asleep.
    (3) Fluid restriction is concerned with limiting the volume of fluid, not the type of fluid.
  * (4) The patient and nurse should make a fluid schedule taking into consideration factors such as periods of wakefulness, number of meals, oral medications, personal preferences, and so on. An appropriate schedule might be ½ the fluid volume between 8 A.M. and 4 P.M. (500 ml), ⅖ of the fluid volume between 4 P.M. and 11 P.M. (400 ml), and the remainder of the fluid (100 ml) during the night.

26.   * (1) This indicates mucus is in the airway; suctioning is necessary to maintain a patent airway because an unconscious patient cannot voluntarily cough.
    (2) Immediate intervention is not necessary because coughing and expectorating are maintaining a patent airway.
    (3) This is an expected response to activity.
    (4) Immediate intervention is unnecessary. While awake, normal respiratory rates are usually between 12 and 20 per minute; when asleep the need for oxygen declines, resulting in a decrease in the respiratory rate and an increase in the depth of respirations.

27.   (1) This would abandon the patient and is not an acceptable intervention; a crying patient needs support, not isolation.
    (2) This supports the patient's need for identity, dignity, and respect, not privacy.
    (3) This supports the patient's right to know what is going to be done and why, not privacy.
  * (4) This provides a personal, secluded environment for a confidential discussion.

28.   (1) This is used for a rectal temperature.
    (2) This is unnecessary; however, daily temperatures should be taken at the same time for comparison purposes. Temperatures usually are highest between 4 and 6 P.M. and lowest between 1 and 4 P.M.
  * (3) Because the machine is used for multiple patients, a probe cover is a medical aseptic technique used to prevent the spread of microorganisms. It provides a barrier between the patient and the machine.
    (4) This is inadequate; a new disposable probe cover should be used for each patient to control the transmission of microorganisms.

29.   (1) Washing should be done in the other direction because it moves secretions and debris away from the urinary meatus, preventing infection.
  * (2) Smegma collects under the foreskin, which must be retracted to permit thorough cleaning.
    (3) A light touch may be too stimulating; a gentle but firm touch is more effective.
    (4) This could injure delicate perineal tissue as well as be too stimulating.

30.   (1) This limits incisional pain and prevents dehiscence.
    (2) Although ambulation increases the respiratory rate, its primary purpose is to prevent circulatory complications such as thrombosis.
  * (3) This helps promote alveolar expansion and facilitates oxygen–carbon dioxide exchange.
    (4) This prevents contractures and circulatory complications.

7 Practice Questions with Answers and Rationales

THE WORLD OF THE PATIENT AND NURSE

This section encompasses factors that influence the role of the nurse and the delivery of health care. Questions address values, ethics, legal aspects of nursing practice, the definition of nursing practice, the steps in the nursing process (assessment, planning, implementation, and evaluation), the responsibilities associated with the management of nursing practice, meeting spiritual needs of patients, patients' rights, the difference between dependent and independent roles of the nurse, supervising the practice of subordinate staff members, the standards of nursing practice, trends in health care, and agencies that provide structure for the delivery of health care.

Questions

1. The patient tells the nurse that her new bathrobe is missing. The nurse's MOST appropriate response would be to:
   (1) Determine if the patient is angry
   (2) Initiate a search for the patient's bathrobe
   (3) Provide an isolation gown that can be used as a robe
   (4) State that it must have gone down with the soiled linen

2. The nurse assigns a nurse aide to a patient who transfers to a chair with a mechanical lift. It has been a long time since the nurse aide used the lift. To ensure the safety of the patient, the nurse should:
   (1) Assign the patient to another nurse aide
   (2) Explain to the nurse aide how to use the lift

    (3) Ask the nurse aide to demonstrate how to use the lift
    (4) Request another care giver to assist with the transfer

3. Which of the following is a dependent activity of the nurse?
    (1) Changing a sterile dressing when soiled
    (2) Assisting with selection of choices on the menu
    (3) Administering oxygen for acute shortness of breath
    (4) Completing documentation about perioperative nursing care

4. The MOST important reason that the nurse must understand the scientific rationale for the actions that constitute a procedure is that the nurse should be able to:
    (1) Implement the procedure safely
    (2) Formulate the nursing care plan
    (3) Document the nursing care given
    (4) Explain the procedure to the patient

5. The nurse observes Mr. Jones going into another patient's room without permission and upsetting the other patient. The nurse's initial response should be to:
    (1) Assist Mr. Jones back to his own room
    (2) Place Mr. Jones in a geri-chair temporarily
    (3) Determine the motivation for Mr. Jones' behavior
    (4) Share the observation about Mr. Jones with the health team

6. Which of the following is the most appropriate activity for a nurse aide?
    (1) Assessing vital signs
    (2) Assisting patients with hygiene
    (3) Monitoring tube feeding machines
    (4) Ambulating postoperative patients

7. On the third day of hospitalization a patient informs the nurse that she would rather bathe at night. To best promote continuity of care, the nurse should:
    (1) Explain that A.M. care is given in the morning
    (2) Verbally inform the other health team members
    (3) Indicate this preference on the nursing care plan
    (4) Encourage her to modify her routine while hospitalized

8. When formulating an assignment for the nurse aide, the nurse should include which of the following tasks?
    (1) Monitoring patients' tube feedings
    (2) Transferring and ambulating patients
    (3) Assessing vital signs and regulating IVs
    (4) Assisting patients with taking medications

9. The charge nurse directs the nurse to do something that is outside the legal role of the nurse. The nurse should:
    (1) Complete the task and grieve later
    (2) Notify the supervisor immediately
    (3) Decline to do the assigned task
    (4) Inform the union representative

10. After a month in the hospital a Jewish patient says she misses lighting her candles on Friday night (Shabbas licht). The MOST therapeutic response would be:
    (1) "It must be difficult to change old habits."
    (2) "Religious traditions have a peaceful effect."
    (3) "I am sorry but that's against the fire code."
    (4) "I will try to arrange it so you can light your candles."

11. Which of the following actions by the nurse would violate patient confidentiality and privacy?
    (1) Writing patient statements in the progress notes
    (2) Interviewing a patient in the presence of others

(3) Presenting the patient's problems at a team conference
(4) Sharing data about a patient at change-of-shift report

12. Mr. Carey has dementia, is verbally and physically abusive, and is paranoid. When providing care, the nurse should always:
(1) Administer care as quickly as possible
(2) Explain everything that is to be done
(3) Tell him what he wants to hear
(4) Tell him how nice he looks

13. When a patient dies, the nurse should begin postmortem care:
(1) After the attending physician has been notified
(2) Once the nursing supervisor has been informed
(3) After significant others have left
(4) As soon as death is pronounced

14. Mr. Alvoir is angry because he cannot perform the activities of daily living by himself. To best reduce his anger, the nurse should:
(1) Disregard his angry behavior
(2) Offer him choices about his care
(3) Gently set limits on his behavior
(4) Encourage him to recognize his limitations

15. Which of the following is a right of patients in a hospital?
(1) Being able to smoke in their room
(2) Refusing treatment ordered by the physician
(3) Requesting meals at the times they prefer
(4) Demanding that they be moved to private rooms

16. Mrs. Fernandez does not like anyone to go into her closet or drawers. When returning hygiene equipment, the nurse should:
(1) Store the equipment on the bedside stand
(2) Allow her to put her equipment in her own drawers
(3) Explain the safety hazard of not putting equipment away
(4) Reassure her that her personal things will not be taken

17. The first task to be completed by the nurse when arriving on the unit for work is to:
(1) Prioritize care to be completed during the shift
(2) Count controlled drugs with the off-going nurse
(3) Make rounds and check the safety of patients
(4) Receive a report on the status of patients

18. When the nurse formulates a nurse aide assignment, the nurse recognizes that the nurse aide job description generally includes which of the following activities?
(1) Ensuring that patients swallow their medications
(2) Reporting unusual gross symptoms to the nurse
(3) Orienting a new nurse aide to the unit
(4) Teaching patients basic self-care

19. The nurse breaks a patients's dentures because of carelessness. What specific legal term applies to his action?
(1) Battery
(2) Assault
(3) Negligence
(4) Malpractice

20. Mrs. Cast is often argumentative and demanding. When planning her care, the nurse's best intervention would be:
(1) Involving her in the decision making
(2) Bringing another staff member as a witness

(3) Accepting her behavior as probably a lifelong pattern
(4) Explaining that the staff would appreciate her cooperation

21. Nurses are required by law to:
    (1) Report situations concerning any form of rape
    (2) Stop at the scene of an accident to give care
    (3) Inform parents if a daughter seeks an abortion
    (4) Notify authorities about instances of child abuse

22. The nurse would have to consider obtaining a consent for surgery from the next of kin when the patient is:
    (1) An extremely elderly woman
    (2) A 16-year-old married woman
    (3) An illiterate 48-year-old man
    (4) A very depressed 55-year-old man

23. The American Nurses Association (ANA) Standards of Nursing Practice are:
    (1) Legal statutes guiding nursing practice
    (2) Step-by-step actions for a nursing procedure
    (3) The requirements for registered nurse licensure
    (4) Policy statements defining the obligations of nurses

24. A patient with dementia needs assistance with hygiene, grooming, eating, and toileting. On discharge from the hospital the agency that would best meet this patient's needs would be:
    (1) A nursing home
    (2) A psychiatric institution
    (3) An adult daycare program
    (4) An outpatient care facility

25. If Miss Susan Jones, a registered nurse, stops at the scene of an accident, she is:
    (1) Provided legal immunity by the Good Samaritan Law
    (2) Meeting the legal trust that accompanies her license
    (3) Held responsible for the care she provides at the scene
    (4) Immune from prosecution because a contract does not exist

26. A voluntary agency is classified as such because it is:
    (1) A health maintenance organization (HMO)
    (2) Supported by volunteer services
    (3) Privately owned and operated
    (4) A nonprofit organization

27. Which of the following is an example of a goal?
    (1) The patient will be fed all meals.
    (2) The patient will be at risk for weight loss.
    (3) The patient will maintain a weight of 140 pounds.
    (4) The patient will need small frequent feedings.

28. Alcoholics Anonymous is classified in which of the following categories?
    (1) Proprietary
    (2) Voluntary
    (3) Official
    (4) Private

29. A nurse says to a patient, "You should get a second opinion because your physician is not the best." The nurse could be sued for:
    (1) Libel
    (2) Assault

(3) Slander
(4) Negligence

30. A nurse's signature on an informed consent for surgery indicates that the:
    (1) Surgeon described the procedure and its risks
    (2) Patient actually signed the consent form
    (3) Patient is informed about his condition
    (4) Surgeon is protected from being sued

31. When obtaining a health history, the nurse identifies that the patient has gained 10 pounds in the last week. When the nurse communicates this information to the physician, the nurse is performing which step in the nursing process?
    (1) Planning
    (2) Analysis
    (3) Assessment
    (4) Evaluation

32. The trend in health care that has received the most attention in the 1990s is:
    (1) Tertiary care
    (2) Early diagnosis
    (3) Health promotion
    (4) Restorative rehabilitation

33. When identifying an excoriated perineal area in the patient with diarrhea, the nurse has performed what step of the nursing process?
    (1) Analysis
    (2) Assessment
    (3) Evaluation
    (4) Implementation

34. The primary purpose of the *National Council Licensure Examination for Nursing* (NCLEX-RN) is to:
    (1) Control nursing
    (2) Verify graduation
    (3) Identify minimal safe practice
    (4) Accredit schools of nursing

35. Which of the following is an example of a patient goal?
    (1) The patient will establish regular bowel habits.
    (2) The patient has a potential for constipation.
    (3) The patient will be toileted every 4 hours.
    (4) The patient needs a commode when toileting.

Rationales

1. (1) This does not address the problem of the missing bathrobe, although the nurse should recognize the resident's right to be angry in this situation.
    * (2) Patients have a right to expect that efforts will be implemented to ensure security for their belongings.
    (3) Although this may be done, it does not address the problem of the missing bathrobe.
    (4) This does not address the feelings of loss, nor is it an attempt to find the robe.

2.   (1) This does not address the nurse aide's need to know how to safely move a patient with a mechanical lift.
      (2) This is unsafe; this teaching method does not take into consideration the need for the nurse aide to practice psychomotor skills associated with this task. Explaining is not enough; a demonstration and return demonstration meeting all the critical elements regarding principles of mechanical lift transfer should be done before a nurse aide can be considered capable of using a mechanical lift safely.
   * (3) Demonstration is the safest way to assess whether the nurse aide has the knowledge and skill to safely transfer a patient using a mechanical lift.
      (4) Another nurse aide should not be held accountable for the care assigned another staff member; the nurse is directly responsible for ensuring that delegated care is safely delivered to patients.

3. * (1) Dependent activities of the nurse are those activities that require a physician's order; this action requires a physician's order.
      (2) Selecting choices of foods offered within a diet is an independent function and does not require a physician's order; however, the type of diet is a dependent function.
      (3) In an emergency the nurse may administer oxygen to a patient experiencing acute shortness of breath until a physician's order can be obtained.
      (4) This is an independent function of the nurse and does not require a physician's order.

4. * (1) Safety of the patient always takes priority; the nurse must perform only those skills that are understood and practiced.
      (2) Patient safety takes priority; however, nurses also need to understand scientific rationales to appropriately plan care.
      (3) The nurse generally does not document the scientific rationale for care given but rather that it was implemented along with the patient's response.
      (4) While it is important to explain all procedures to the patient, safety takes priority; nurses need to have a strong scientific foundation to provide safe care.

5. * (1) Patients have a right to privacy and security for themselves and their belonging; returning him to his room removes him from the other patient's room.
      (2) Restraining a resident in situations other than for their own physical safety and without a physician's order is illegal.
      (3) First the patient needs to be removed from the other patient's room; once in his own room the nurse can explore the motivation for the behavior.
      (4) This does not address the immediate need to remove the patient from the room of another; once the behavior is addressed then it can be communicated.

6.   (1) This requires professional nursing judgment; the nurse is educationally prepared to determine the significance of vital sign measurements, not the nurse aide.
   * (2) Nurse aides are trained to provide basic hygiene measures under the direction of a nurse.
      (3) It is not legal for a nurse aide to monitor tube feedings; this action is within the legal practice of nursing, not nurse aide practice.
      (4) Nurses should ambulate postoperative patients; nurses have the knowledge to analyze a patient's response to ambulating postoperatively. Nurse aides ambulate patients with simple, noncomplex needs.

7.   (1) Hygiene care is not only done in the morning; care should be individualized.
   (2) This would not provide a written plan of care for nurses to refer to when implementing nursing care.
* (3) This provides for a written plan of care of what should be done for the patient; it supports communication among nurses, contributes to continuity, and individualizes care.
   (4) This is not necessary; care should be individualized and communicated via a nursing care plan.

8.   (1) This is the legal responsibility of the nurse, not the nurse aide.
* (2) Nurse aides are responsible for meeting patients' basic activities of daily living (ADL) needs under the supervision of the nurse; transfer and ambulation are basic ADL.
   (3) Same as #1.
   (4) Same as #1.

9.   (1) Nurses should perform only those tasks that they are licensed to perform.
   (2) The first action should be to respectfully decline to do the task; the nurse should notify the supervisor if the charge nurse continues to insist that the task be performed.
* (3) Performing a task that is outside the legal definition of the nurse is illegal; a nurse has the responsibility to refuse to follow an order that is illegal.
   (4) Same as #2; a union representative is usually notified in the event that the supervisor threatens the nurse (not all agencies are unionized).

10.   (1) This fails to recognize the religious significance of lighting candles and does not support the patient's need to perform this religious activity.
   (2) This ignores the patient's need to experience the spiritual activity of lighting the candles.
   (3) This is untrue; if performed under supervision, it can be safely done.
* (4) Religious rituals support spiritual and emotional needs and should be encouraged when they comfort the patient.

11.   (1) This is an acceptable practice; the purpose of progress notes is to share and communicate data about the patient.
* (2) This violates confidentiality; others may overhear information that should be kept confidential.
   (3) This is an acceptable practice; a team conference enables professionals to share and communicate important information about patients.
   (4) This is an appropriate practice; sharing information at report notifies the nurses of the patient's changing status.

12.   (1) This does not address the right of the patient to know what is being done and why; rushing may increase the patient's anxiety.
* (2) This supports every patient's right to know what care is being given and why; understanding increases compliance; this is especially important with people who are paranoid.
   (3) This is patronizing; when patients feel they are being humored, trust deteriorates.
   (4) This may not be true; trust is based on honesty.

13.   (1) Postmortem care should not begin until after death is pronounced and the family has an opportunity to make a last visit.
   (2) Same as #1.

* (3) This allows the family members time to make a last visit before the body is prepared for transfer to a mortuary.

(4) This does not recognize the right of the family to see the deceased one last time prior to postmortem care.

14. (1) Behavior should not be disregarded or ignored; all behavior has meaning and requires recognition.

* (2) Making decisions puts the patient in control and supports feelings of independence.

(3) This will only make the patient more angry because it is a controlling intervention.

(4) This will only intensify feelings of dependence.

15. (1) Some hospitals provide designated smoking areas. The Joint Commission on Accreditation of Healthcare Organizations, the agency responsible for accrediting hospitals, has identified a new standard to be effective January 1, 1993, which states that as of this date, health care organizations seeking Joint Commission accreditation will be required to be "smoke free."

* (2) The patient has a right to refuse care against medical advice; the physician needs to explain to the patient the risks involved in lack of treatment.

(3) Meals are generally scheduled during regular mealtimes. It is impractical to serve meals any time a patient prefers; however, if a special need arises, the nurse generally should attempt to individualize care.

(4) A private room is generally a privilege, not a right, that is provided for at extra expense; it is not automatically provided on demand. However, a patient requiring isolation may be transferred to a private room.

16. (1) This does not support the patient's need to be in control of the immediate environment; equipment should be stored appropriately to protect it from pathogens in the environment.

* (2) This supports the patient's right to control personal space.

(3) Logic does not reduce paranoid behavior; the patient needs to feel in control, and this action does not support this need.

(4) Same as #3.

17. (1) Before the nurse can prioritize care, the nurse must first receive report to know about each patient's status.

(2) Communicating about the status of patients should be the first order of business upon arrival; after report, controlled drugs can be counted.

(3) Rounds are implemented after report. The nurse first needs to know the status of the patients; report provides baseline data about patients that are needed before additional assessments can be planned. Some hospitals have walking rounds where report and assessment of patients are simultaneously conducted.

* (4) Before care can be planned and implemented, the nurse needs to know the condition and immediate needs of the patients.

18. (1) This is a legal responsibility of the nurse; it is illegal for the nurse aide to give drugs, even under the supervision of the nurse.

* (2) The nurse aide is trained to identify major abnormal signs and symptoms and to notify the nurse when a sign is outside the normal range or is changed from the patient's baseline; the nurse then completes a professional assessment of the patient's condition.

(3) A nurse aide should always work under the direct guidance and supervision of a nurse, not another nurse aide.

(4) Teaching requires a strong scientific knowledge base and an ability to utilize scientific teaching-learning principles when planning and implementing an educational plan; the nurse aide is not prepared for this responsibility.

19. (1) Battery is the purposeful, angry, or negligent touching of a patient without consent.

(2) Assault is an act intended to provoke fear in a patient.

 * (3) Negligence occurs when the nurse's actions do not meet appropriate standards and result in injury to another; negligence can occur with acts of omission or commission.

(4) Malpractice is misconduct performed in professional practice that results in harm to another.

20. * (1) The patient is the center of the health team and has a right to be involved in the decision making concerning care; this individualizes care and promotes self-esteem.

(2) This is a defensive response. All behavior has meaning; the nurse should initially accept the behavior, involve the patient, and identify the reason for the behavior.

(3) This is an assumption; many people cope with anxiety by being argumentative and demanding. This behavior may be an attempt to gain control in a situation where the individual feels out of control.

(4) This is judgmental and takes away the patient's coping mechanism.

21. (1) It is the responsibility of the injured person to report an incident of rape.

(2) This is an ethical responsibility, not a legal requirement.

(3) In June 1992 the Supreme Court of the United States upheld the constitutional right of a woman to control her own body to the extent that she can abort a fetus in the early stages of pregnancy. However, the decision stipulated that each state may legislate its own reasonable restrictions. It is likely that some states will require parental notification if the woman seeking an abortion is a minor. Notification should not be confused with consent. Also, the question does not indicate that the daughter is a minor.

 * (4) It is a law that requires professionals, such as teachers, certain health care professionals, and social workers, to report suspicions of child abuse to the authorities.

22. (1) The ability to understand the surgery and its implications and alternatives is related to emotional and mental stability, not age.

(2) An under-legal-age person with a valid marriage certificate can sign a surgical consent form.

(3) A patient who is illiterate can sign by making a mark on the consent form; the nurse is a witness to attest that the mark was made by the patient.

 * (4) A patient must be mentally and emotionally competent to sign a surgical consent form; depression can interfere with cognitive processes and comprehension.

23. (1) Legal statutes are laws created by elected legislative bodies; they are not nursing standards.

(2) This is a procedure or protocol, not a standard of practice.

(3) Although the requirements for licensure vary slightly among states, most licensing acts require a specified level of education and the passing of a special examination.

* (4) The American Nurses' Association (ANA) has general resolutions that recommend the responsibilities and obligations of nurses; these standards help determine if a nurse has acted as any prudent reasonable nurse would with a similar education, experiential background, and environment.

24. * (1) This patient needs long-term nursing care as well as 24-hour supervision.
(2) This type of a setting would be inappropriate for this patient; patients with dementia need supportive care for the rest of their lives. Psychiatric settings today provide acute care services for mentally ill patients.
(3) There are no data that indicate the support of a family or the ability to provide self-care when not at the daycare center; most daycare programs function 5 days a week from 8 A.M. until 6 P.M. to assist working family members.
(4) These facilities usually provide acute care services, not long-term nursing care or 24-hour supervision.

25. (1) It does not provide legal immunity; the nurse can still be held accountable for gross departure from acceptable standards of practice or willful wrongdoing.
(2) Assistance at the scene of an accident is an ethical, not a legal, duty.
* (3) Nurses are responsible for their own actions, and the care provided must be what any reasonably prudent nurse would do under similar circumstances.
(4) A contract does not have to exist for a nurse to commit negligence.

26. (1) Health maintenance organizations are usually proprietary agencies that attempt to make a profit.
(2) Although volunteers serve as helpers and supporters to voluntary agencies, this is not the reason for the classification; voluntary agencies are nonprofit organizations.
(3) This would be a proprietary agency.
* (4) Voluntary agencies may not make a profit; any money made must be applied to operating expenses and provision of services.

27. (1) This is an intervention, not a goal.
(2) This is part of a problem statement, not a goal.
* (3) This is a goal statement that is specific, measurable, and contains a time frame; *maintain* implies continuously.
(4) This is a statement that identifies a need or intervention in response to an identified problem, not a goal.

28. (1) Proprietary agencies are privately owned and operated to make a profit.
* (2) Alcoholics Anonymous (AA) is a voluntary organization; voluntary agencies are not-for-profit and rely on professional and lay volunteers, in addition to a paid staff, to meet a specific identified health need.
(3) Official health agencies are supported by local, state, and national taxes and are designed to meet a specific health need on the local, state, or national level.
(4) Same as #1.

29. (1) This is defamation of character via print, writing, or pictures, not spoken words.
(2) This is an attempt or threat to touch another person unjustifiably.

* (3) This is defamation of character by spoken words.
  (4) Negligence is the omission to do something a reasonably prudent nurse would do under similar circumstances or the commission of an act that a reasonably prudent nurse would not do under similar circumstances.

30. (1) The nurse's signature does not document that the physician described the procedure and its risks; the patient's signature documents that the procedure and its risks are understood.
* (2) The nurse only witnesses the patient's signature.
  (3) The nurse only witnesses the patient's signature and examines the document for the correct date and time; the nurse's signature does not document that the patient was properly informed.
  (4) This is untrue; reasonable prudent practice protects the surgeon from being sued.

31. (1) Planning is involved with setting goals, establishing priorities, identifying expected outcomes, identifying interventions designed to achieve goals and outcomes, modifying the plan as necessary, and collaborating with other health team members to ensure that care is coordinated. Planning does not include the communication of data collected during assessment.
  (2) Analysis is involved with the interpretation of data, collection of additional data, identification and communication of nursing diagnoses, and the assurance that the patient's health care needs are appropriately met. Analysis does not include the communication of data collected during the assessment phase of the nursing process.
* (3) Communicating important assessment data to other health team members is a component of the assessment phase of the nursing process.
  (4) Evaluation is involved with identifying a patient's response to care, comparing a patient's actual responses to the expected outcomes, analyzing factors that affected the actual outcomes for the purpose of drawing conclusions about the success or failure of specific nursing activities, and modifying the nursing care plan when necessary. Evaluation does not include the communication of data collected during the assessment phase.

32. (1) *Tertiary care* involves helping patients adapt to limitations caused by illness.
  (2) Early diagnosis and treatment to prevent complications of illness are *secondary care.*
* (3) This is *primary care;* health promotion activities, such as exercise programs and low-cholesterol diets, assist patients to maintain their present levels of health or enhance their health in the future. *Primary care* has received increased importance in the 1990s.
  (4) This is *tertiary care.*

33. (1) In the analysis step of the nursing process, the nurse interprets data, determines the significance of data, and formulates a nursing diagnosis.
* (2) Observation of human responses is part of the assessment phase of the nursing process; assessment involves collecting, verifying, clustering, and communicating objective and subjective data.
  (3) Evaluation involves determining patient responses to nursing interventions, identifying if goals and outcomes are met, and revising the nursing care plan when necessary.
  (4) Implementation involves carrying out the nursing care plan and documenting the care provided.

34.   (1) Nurse practice acts define and control the licensure and practice of nursing in each state, not NCLEX-RN.

  (2) A degree or diploma verifies that the student has met the criteria for graduation from the granting institution, not NCLEX-RN

* (3) The NCLEX-RN exam is designed to identify whether a candidate has met a minimum level of performance to safely practice as a licensed registered nurse.

  (4) The National League for Nursing (NLN) and the state boards of nursing have established standards that must be met in order for an associate degree, diploma, or baccalaureate degree program to be accredited.

35. * (1) This is a goal because it identifies a desired patient outcome or change in patient behavior.

  (2) This is the problem statement part of a nursing diagnosis; it is the phrase that precedes the words "related to" in a nursing diagnosis.

  (3) This is a planned intervention.

  (4) This is a patient need that directly influences the planned intervention.

COMMON THEORIES RELATED TO MEETING PATIENTS' BASIC HUMAN NEEDS

This section encompasses questions related to the work of theorists such as Maslow, Kübler-Ross, Selye, and Erickson. It also includes questions related to principles of teaching, growth and development, types of stresses, and the definition of health.

Questions

1. Of the following human needs identified by Maslow, which is the *most* basic?
   (1) Physiological needs
   (2) Belonging needs
   (3) Security needs
   (4) Safety needs

2. To ensure that a patient understands the content of a teaching session, the nurse should:
   (1) Ask the patient what was learned
   (2) Speak distinctly when giving directions
   (3) Speak slowly when talking with the patient
   (4) Use simple vocabulary and sentence structure

3. To meet a patient's basic physiological need according to Maslow's hierarchy of needs, the nurse should:
   (1) Pull the curtain when the patient is on a bedpan
   (2) Maintain the patient in functional alignment
   (3) Respond to the call light immediately
   (4) Raise both side rails on the bed

4. A developmental task of the elderly identified by Erickson is:
   (1) Assisting grown children
   (2) Reconciling one's life
   (3) Establishing trust
   (4) Becoming dependent

5. A mentally disadvantaged (retarded) adult patient is learning self-care. To increase learning, the nurse should:
   (1) Verbally recognize when goals are met
   (2) Use candy as a reward when goals are met
   (3) Set a variety of short-term goals to be met
   (4) Disregard the behavior when goals are not met

6. The following action that would meet a patient's basic physiological need is:
   (1) Conversing with the patient
   (2) Raising the side rails
   (3) Explaining procedures
   (4) Providing a bed bath

7. The process of growth and development can generally be described as:
   (1) Plodding
   (2) Unique
   (3) Simple
   (4) Even

8. In relation to Erickson's developmental theory, a question that could be asked that relates to the task of the school-age child is:
   (1) "Who am I?"
   (2) "What can I do?"
   (3) "Who can I trust?"
   (4) "What have I done?"

9. A patient draws pictures and hangs them in his room. The basic human need being met by this action is:
   (1) Physiological
   (2) Self-esteem
   (3) Security
   (4) Love

10. Growth and development follows a pattern that:
    (1) Is unpredictable
    (2) Relies on motivation
    (3) Is based on the previous step
    (4) Depends on personal strengths

11. According to Erikson's developmental theory, a statement that can be associated with the task of generativity versus stagnation is:
    (1) "I am pleased with the decisions I have made."
    (2) "I will be getting married next week."
    (3) "I enjoy mentoring the new employees."
    (4) "I want to do it myself."

12. A sunburn is considered a:
    (1) Chemical stress
    (2) Physical stress
    (3) Physiological stress
    (4) Microbiological stress

13. According to Erikson, an event that would support the developmental tasks associated with the stage of middle adulthood would be:
    (1) Getting married
    (2) Becoming a parent
    (3) Retiring from work
    (4) Experiencing menopause

14. Infants have very light yellow urine because they:
    (1) Ingest just fluids
    (2) Cannot control urination
    (3) Are unable to concentrate urine
    (4) Urinate more frequently than adults

15. An activity that would promote successful completion of the struggle associated with young adulthood would be:
    (1) Going on a date
    (2) Raising children
    (3) Promoting a cause
    (4) Sharing knowledge

16. When planning to teach colostomy care to a young adult male who has just had a temporary colostomy, the nurse should initially:
    (1) Identify the patient's interest in self-care
    (2) Determine the patient's usual bowel habits
    (3) Reinforce that the colostomy is temporary
    (4) Establish goals for the teaching plan

17. According to Maslow, when planning care for several patients, the nurse should first assist the patient who needs to:
    (1) Void
    (2) Talk
    (3) Walk
    (4) Know

18. An activity that supports the developmental task of the adolescent would be:
    (1) Reading a book
    (2) Learning how to use a computer
    (3) Helping parents with household chores
    (4) Attending a high school basketball game

19. When considering definitions about health, one concept that is basic to most definitions is that health is:
    (1) Absence of disease
    (2) A progressive state
    (3) Relative to one's value system
    (4) An extreme of the health-illness continuum

20. Which word best describes feelings associated with an infant in Erikson's stage of trust versus mistrust?
    (1) Me
    (2) We
    (3) You
    (4) They

21. According to Maslow's hierarchy of needs, which of the following would most clearly demonstrate physiological needs as a priority?
    (1) Trauma
    (2) Puberty
    (3) Menopause
    (4) Restraints

22. Considering theories about stress, which of the following generally precipitates the highest degree of stress?
    (1) Retirement
    (2) Relocation

(3) Pregnancy
(4) Marriage

23. When collecting information to prepare a teaching plan in the cognitive domain, the nurse asks the patient:
(1) "Can you measure a serum glucose level?"
(2) "What do you know about diabetes mellitus?"
(3) "How do you feel about having diabetes melitus?"
(4) "Are you able to perform a subcutaneous injection?"

24. Which word best reflects the type of play associated with Erikson's stage of initiative versus guilt?
(1) Me
(2) Us
(3) You
(4) Them

25. The elderly tend to have higher blood pressures because older people have:
(1) Vessels that are less elastic
(2) Stressful lifestyle changes
(3) Blood that is thicker
(4) Hearts that are aging

26. The most appropriate way to teach a patient about self-injection with insulin would be through a:
(1) Demonstration
(2) Discussion
(3) Movie
(4) Book

27. According to Maslow's hierarchy of needs, which of the needs listed below takes priority?
(1) Security
(2) Belonging
(3) Self-esteem
(4) Self-actualization

28. An adult has a sense of inadequacy and inferiority at work. One could say that this person had the most difficulty resolving the conflict associated with which of the following developmental ages?
(1) Birth to 1 year
(2) 4 to 8 years
(3) 8 to 12 years
(4) 13 to 20 years

29. The stress of air pollution caused by wood burning fireplaces in the home can be classified as a:
(1) Chemical stress
(2) Physical stress
(3) Physiological stress
(4) Microbiological stress

30. Which of the following is most relevant when predicting success of a teaching program regarding the learning of a skill?
(1) The learner's cognitive ability
(2) The extent of family support
(3) The interest of the learner
(4) The amount of reinforcement

Rationales

1. * (1) These are most basic; oxygen, food, fluid, rest, sleep, and elimination are basic for life.
      (2) This need is ranked third after physiological and safety-security needs and before self-actualization.
      (3) This need is ranked second after physiological needs and before love and belonging.
      (4) Same as #3.

2. * (1) Seeking feedback enables the caregiver to know whether or not the message was understood as intended.
      (2) This helps to send a clearer message, but it does not inform the sender whether the receiver understood the message.
      (3) Same as #2.
      (4) Same as #2.

3.   (1) This supports the need for self-esteem; it provides for privacy.
    * (2) This supports a basic physiological need; this reduces physical strain and potential injury to joints, muscles, ligaments, and tendons and can prevent the formation of contractures.
      (3) This supports the need for security and safety; patients need to know that help is immediately available when needed.
      (4) This supports the need for safety and security; bed rails prevent a patient from falling out of bed.

4.   (1) Middle-aged adults may help grown children; this is usually a task of this age group.
    * (2) The elderly need to come to terms with the fact that the end of life is near; reviewing one's life is a step in this process.
      (3) An infant needs to develop trust; this is the major task of this age.
      (4) Dependency is not a task for which one strives; dependency results if an 8- to 12-year-old is unable to resolve the conflict of industry versus inferiority.

5. * (1) This would support feelings of self-esteem and independence; it provides external reinforcement and promotes internal reinforcement.
      (2) Candy is not good for health; praise is a more acceptable reward.
      (3) A mentally disadvantaged person generally can focus on only one goal at a time; several goals may be overwhelming.
      (4) A patient's behavior should never be disregarded; all behavior should be addressed in a nonjudgmental and supportive manner.

6.   (1) This relates to the need for love and belonging, the third level in Maslow's hierarchy of needs.
      (2) This relates to the need for safety and security, the second level in Maslow's hierarchy of needs.
      (3) This relates to the need for safety and security; patients have a right to know what is happening to them and why.
    * (4) This supports the physiological need to be clean and is related to the first level, physical needs, in Maslow's hierarchy of needs.

7.   (1) Some stages are faster and some are slower.
    * (2) While a general pattern is followed, each individual grows and develops at a different rate or extent.

      (3) This is an extremely complex process based on many influencing variables.

      (4) Just the opposite; some states are faster and some are slower depending on the stage and the individual.

8.   (1) This involves the conflict of identify versus role confusion; the person aged 13 to 20 years seeks to develop peer relationships, defines goals, selects a vocation, gains independence, and seeks identity.

  * (2) This involves the conflict of industry versus inferiority; the child of 6 to 12 years is developing a sense of competence and perseverance.

      (3) This involves the conflict of trust versus mistrust. During the first year the infant depends on others to meet basic needs; the infant develops trust if these needs are met in a comfortable and predictable manner.

      (4) This involves the conflict of integrity versus despair; the person aged 60 years or more struggles to feel a sense of worth about past experiences and goals achieved and seeks a sense of integrity.

9.   (1) "Physiological" relates to meeting basic physical needs such as the need for oxygen, food, water, rest, sleep, and elimination, not self-esteem.

  * (2) The situation illustrated in the item meets self-esteem needs; control, self-respect, and competence are reflected when a person hangs self-made pictures in a room for the enjoyment of self and others.

      (3) "Security" refers to shelter, clothing, and the need to feel comfortable with the rules of the society, community, and hospital.

      (4) "Love" refers to the need for bonds of affection and a sense of belonging.

10.   (1) While growth and development progress through some stages slower or faster than others, they still follow a basic predictable pattern.

      (2) Motivation may influence the achievement of tasks in some stages of growth and development; however, growth and development do not rely on motivation.

  * (3) Success or failure of task achievement in one stage of development influences succeeding stages; failure to resolve a crisis at one stage damages the ego which makes the resolution of the following stages more difficult.

      (4) Personal strengths may assist a person to more easily achieve a particular developmental task; however, growth and development do not depend on personal strengths.

11.   (1) This is stage 8; this is the conflict of integrity versus despair. The person aged 60 years or more struggles to feel a sense of worth about past experiences and goals achieved and seeks a sense of integrity.

      (2) This is stage 6; this is the conflict of intimacy and solidarity versus isolation. The young adult 20 to 30 years old seeks to select a partner for a life relationship.

  * (3) This is stage 7; this is a conflict of generativity versus self-absorption. The person 30 to 60 years old is interested in guiding younger individuals.

      (4) This is stage 2; it is the conflict of autonomy versus shame and doubt. The 2- to 4-year-old seeks a balance between independence and dependence and attempts to achieve autonomy.

12.   (1) Chemical stresses relate to toxic substances such as acids, alkalies, drugs, and exogenous hormones.

  * (2) Physical stresses are stresses from outside the body and include light, environmental temperature, sound, pressure, motion, gravity, and electricity.

(3) Physiological stresses are disturbances in structure or function of any tissue, organ, or system within the body.

(4) Microbiological stresses are organisms such as bacteria, viruses, fungi, or parasites that can cause disease.

13.   (1) This is most often associated with young adulthood, intimacy versus isolation.

* (2) Concerns for the family and next generation are associated with middle adulthood, generativity versus self-absorption.

(3) This is associated with the older adult, integrity versus despair.

(4) Menopause is not associated with any developmental task according to Erikson; Erikson's theory is a psychosocial developmental theory based on the process of socialization, not physiologic events.

14.   (1) Infants void very light yellow urine because they are unable to concentrate urine and reabsorb water efficiently, not because they only ingest fluids.

(2) Although true because infants have not developed neuromuscular control of urination, the inability to voluntarily control micturition has no impact on the color of urine voided.

* (3) An infant's kidneys are unable to concentrate urine and reabsorb water efficiently; when the body is too immature to concentrate urine, urine will be diluted and very light yellow in color.

(4) Infants urinate more frequently than adults because their bladders are smaller and they can only retain a small volume of urine in comparison to an adult. Also because infants cannot concentrate urine and reabsorb water efficiently, they void a larger percentage of urine per day in comparison to an adult; frequency is not related to the color of urine.

15.   * (1) The developmental task of the young adult is the establishment of intimacy with a relationship partner.

(2) This is related to the developmental task of generativity associated with middle adulthood.

(3) Same as #2.

(4) Same as #2.

16.   * (1) Determining the patient's readiness for learning and point of reference are the priorities.

(2) This would be done after a readiness for learning is established.

(3) Same as #2.

(4) Same as #2.

17.   * (1) When setting priorities, usually the most basic physiologic needs must be met first.

(2) Although important, basic physiologic needs must be met first.

(3) Same as #2.

(4) Same as #2.

18.   (1) Middle childhood (6 to 12 years) is concerned with developing fundamental skills in reading, writing, calculating, and using a computer; the school-age child is very industrious.

(2) Same as #1.

(3) The childhood years are related to helping behaviors; 3- to 5-year-olds like to imitate parents, and 6- to 12-year-olds are developing appropriate social roles.
* (4) Adolescents are concerned with developing new and more mature relationships with their peers; adolescents tend to associate with age-mates rather than parents.

19. (1) The World Health Organization's definition of health is, "A state of complete physical, mental and social well being, and not merely the absence of disease or infirmity"; some people who have a chronic illness consider themselves healthy because they are able to function independently.
(2) Health is on a continuum rather than progressive; movement can occur up or down the continuum, not only in one direction.
* (3) A definition of health is highly individualized; it is based on each person's own experiences, values and perceptions. Health can mean different things to each individual; people tend to define health based on the presence or absence of symptoms, perceptions of how they feel, and the capacity to function on a daily basis.
(4) While high-level wellness is one extreme of the health-illness continuum and severe illness the other, where one plots a position on the continuum is based on the individual's value system. An individual's perception of health is based on one's physical, emotional, social, mental, and spiritual sense of wellness.

20. * (1) The infant is very egocentric and is unaware of boundaries between the self and others; the infant is concerned with needs being immediately met.
(2) The infant has not identified the difference between the self and others.
(3) Same as #2.
(4) Same as #2.

21. * (1) Trauma can be life threatening and interfere with basic physiological functioning.
(2) Although there are physiologic changes associated with the growth spurt and development of secondary sexual characteristics during puberty, self-identity and self-esteem often take priority at this time.
(3) Although there are physiological changes associated with menopause, love, self-esteem, or self-actualization often are the priorities at this time.
(4) Restraints meet safety and security needs because they protect the patient from harm.

22. (1) Stress units for life events have been determined based on the readjustment required by an individual to adapt to a particular situation or event; the mean stress unit for retirement is 45 and is less than marriage, which is 50.
(2) The mean stress unit for a change in residence is 20.
(3) The mean stress unit for pregnancy is 40.
* (4) The mean stress unit for marriage is 50, which is higher than the other options presented.

23. (1) This is the psychomotor domain because it involves a skill.
* (2) This is the cognitive domain because it deals with information and knowledge.
(3) This is the affective domain because it relates to feelings.
(4) Same as #1.

24. (1) The 2- to 4-year-old, during the conflict of autonomy versus shame and doubt, strives to develop a sense of autonomy and focuses on "me." Also, an infant, during the conflict of trust versus mistrust, is egocentric and is concerned with "me."
  * (2) The child, age 4 to 8, during the conflict of initiative versus guilt, strives to adjust to social spheres outside the home. The child begins to evolve as a social being seeking relationships with a small number of peers with a focus on "us."
   (3) The young adult, age 20 to 30, during the conflict of intimacy and solidarity versus isolation, strives among other tasks to select a relationship partner. A relationship partner in one's life is the important "you."
   (4) The school-age child, 8 through 12 years, during the conflict of industry versus inferiority, strives to become a productive group member; the school-age child joins a "gang," and recognizes the differences of others or "them."

25. * (1) Vascular changes and the accumulation of sclerotic plaques along the walls of vessels make them more rigid.
   (2) This is a generalization which may or may not be true depending on the individual; the older adult will have physical, cognitive, and social changes, and how the person perceives them and adapts to them will determine if the lifestyle is stressful.
   (3) High blood pressure in the elderly is generally caused by smoking, obesity, lack of exercise, and stress, not blood that is thicker.
   (4) A decreased contractile strength of the myocardium results in a decreased cardiac output, which the body compensates for by increasing the heart rate, not the blood pressure.

26. * (1) The opportunity to observe and manipulate the equipment promotes learning a skill; this uses a variety of senses such as sight, hearing, and touch. It is most useful in the psychomotor domain.
   (2) Learning via discussion is appropriate for the cognitive and affective domains.
   (3) Although this can be used for learning a psychomotor skill, it is not as effective as demonstration and return demonstration; it is more appropriate for leaning in the cognitive domain.
   (4) Same as #3.

27. * (1) Safety and security needs, second-level needs according to Maslow, occur after basic physiological needs and before the need for love and belonging; people need to feel physically and emotionally safe.
   (2) This third-level need according to Maslow occurs after safety and security needs; a bond of affection is necessary for well-being.
   (3) This fourth-level need according to Maslow occurs after love and belonging needs; people need to feel competent and respected.
   (4) This is the fifth and final level according to Maslow; maximizing abilities and feeling content within the self are necessary for self-satisfaction.

28. (1) Birth to 1 year of age is concerned with resolving the conflict of trust versus mistrust, not industry versus inferiority.
   (2) During the ages of 4 to 8 years the child is concerned with resolving the conflict of initiative versus guilt, not industry versus inferiority.

* (3) During the ages of 8 to 12 years, the child is concerned with resolving the conflict of industry versus inferiority; when a child is unable to develop physical, social, or cognitive skills well enough to perceive oneself as competent, the child feels inadequate. These feelings of inferiority can be carried throughout adulthood.

(4) During the ages of 13 to 20 years, the child is concerned with resolving the conflict of identity versus role confusion, not industry versus inferiority.

29. * (1) Burning wood releases toxic substances and gases into the air which are considered chemical stresses; acids, alkalies, drugs, and exogenous hormones are also considered chemical stresses.

(2) Air pollution is a chemical stress, not a physical stress; physical stresses include temperature, sound, pressure, light, motion, gravity, and electricity.

(3) Air pollution is a chemical stress, not a physiological stress; disturbances in structure or function of any tissue, organ, or system of the body are considered physiological stresses.

(4) Air pollution is a chemical stress, not a microbiological stress; bacteria, viruses, fungi, and parasites are considered microbiological stresses.

30. (1) Although a teaching program must be designed within the patient's developmental and cognitive abilities, it is useless unless the patient recognizes the value of what is to be learned and has a desire to learn.

(2) Although this is important, the patient's interest and readiness to learn are the priorities for the successful learning of a skill; some patients do not have a family support system.

* (3) The motivation of the learner to acquire new attitudes, information, or skills is the most important component for successful learning; motivation exists when the learner recognizes the future benefits of learning.

(4) Although this is important, self-motivation is the most significant factor in learning.

COMMUNICATION AND MEETING PATIENTS' EMOTIONAL NEEDS

This section encompasses questions related to assessing and meeting patients' sociocultural, psychological, and spiritual needs. It includes questions that focus on the principles of communication, communication skills, interventions that support emotional needs, and communicating with the confused or disoriented patient. Additional questions focus on patterns of behavior in response to illness, nursing interventions that assist patients to adapt to illness, caring for the dying patient's emotional needs, defense mechanisms, and responding to the crying patient.

Questions

1. A nurse will be going on vacation. To involve the patient in the excitement, what is the *best* thing the nurse should say?
   (1) "Let me tell you about the plans for my vacation."
   (2) "Tell me about some of your past vacations."
   (3) "I'll bring the brochures for you to see."
   (4) "What do you think about vacations?"

2. A patient's son has just died. The patient states, "I can't believe that I have lost my son. Can you believe it?" The nurse's BEST response is to:
   (1) Touch her hand and say, "I am very sorry."
   (2) Say, "It is sad. I can't believe it either."
   (3) Leave the room and allow her to grieve privately.
   (4) Encourage a family member to stay and provide support.

3. Which of the following nursing interventions would be least effective in meeting a patient's psychosocial needs?
   (1) Addressing a patient by name
   (2) Assisting a patient with meals
   (3) Identifying achievement of goals
   (4) Explaining care prior to its being given

4. Which of the following is a true statement about communication?
   (1) A patient with expressive aphasia cannot communicate.
   (2) Nurses' notes are a form of nonverbal communication.
   (3) Touch has various meanings to different people.
   (4) Words have the same meaning for all people.

5. The nurse recognizes that a usually talkative patient is withdrawn. The nurse's *best* response would be:
   (1) "Something seems to be bothering you."
   (2) "Why are you so withdrawn today?"
   (3) "Tell me what you're upset about."
   (4) "You are very quiet today."

6. Mrs. Anderson's husband died 1 week ago. When talking about him, she begins to cry. The nurse's best response would be to:
   (1) Leave her alone to provide privacy
   (2) Encourage her to get grief counseling
   (3) Say, "Things will get better as time passes."
   (4) State, "This must be a very difficult time for you."

7. Mr. Murray has been verbally aggressive toward the nurses. One afternoon he starts to shout at another patient in the lounge. The best statement by the nurse would be:
   (1) "Stop what you are doing."
   (2) "Let's go talk in your room."
   (3) "Please sit down and be calm."
   (4) "What seems to be the problem?"

8. Mrs. Michael is being discharged to a nursing home. While preparing the discharge summary, the patient says, "I feel that nobody cares about me." The nurse's *best* response would be:
   (1) "You sound angry at your family."
   (2) "You feel as though nobody cares?"
   (3) "We all care about you and are concerned."
   (4) "Your family doesn't have the skills to care for you."

9. Mrs. Brown is 59 years old, becomes upset whenever anyone mentions her upcoming birthday, and does not want to talk about age. The nurse recognizes this behavior as:
   (1) Denial
   (2) Sorrow
   (3) Loneliness
   (4) Suppression

10. Mrs. Adams who is usually verbal appears sad and withdrawn. The nurse should:
    (1) Describe the patient's behavior to her
    (2) Continue to observe the patient's behavior

(3) Ensure that the patient has time to be alone
(4) Attempt to engage the patient in cheerful conversation

11. When administering care to Mrs. Polski, she talks about her children when they were young and states, "I was a very strict mother." A response by the nurse that reflects the use of the technique of paraphrasing would be:
(1) "It must have been difficult to be a disciplinarian."
(2) "Sometimes we are sorry for our past behaviors."
(3) "You believe you were a firm parent."
(4) "You were a very strict mother."

12. A terminal patient appears sad and withdrawn. The nurse should respond by being:
(1) Demonstrative
(2) Cheerful
(3) Present
(4) Aloof

13. A patient with a chronic illness is depressed. Which of the following behaviors would support this conclusion?
(1) Wishing to attend a nephew's wedding
(2) Evading activities of daily living
(3) Seeking second medical opinions
(4) Being sarcastic to care givers

14. Mr. Sherman, who has been withdrawn, says, "When I have the opportunity, I am going to commit suicide." The *best* response by the nurse would be:
(1) "You have a lovely wife. She needs you."
(2) "Let's explore the reasons you have for living."
(3) "You must feel overwhelmed to want to kill yourself."
(4) "Suicide does not solve problems. Tell me what is wrong."

15. A patient who is hard of hearing tells the nurse he cannot hear what people say to him. The nurse should:
(1) Shout to him with a loud voice in the better ear
(2) Ask questions that require a yes or no answer
(3) Provide pencil and paper for communication
(4) Encourage him to use gestures when talking

16. A patient is confused and disoriented. The route of communication used by the nurse that would be most effective would be:
(1) Touch
(2) Writing
(3) Talking
(4) Pictures

17. A patient asks for advice regarding a personal problem. The *most* appropriate response by the nurse would be to:
(1) Explain that nurses are not permitted to give advice
(2) Offer an opinion after listening to the patient
(3) Encourage the patient to speak with her family
(4) Ask the patient what she thinks she should do

18. Mr. Kolt is crying. The best response by the nurse is:
(1) "Sometimes it helps to talk about it."
(2) "I hope things will get better by tomorrow."
(3) "Deep breathing may help you regain control."
(4) "Crying helps because it gets it out of your system."

19. A dying patient is withdrawn and depressed. The action by the nurse that would be most therapeutic would be:
    (1) Assisting him in focusing on positive thoughts
    (2) Explaining that he still can accomplish goals
    (3) Accepting his behavioral adaptation
    (4) Offering advice when appropriate

20. The sense that is most important to a patient who appears to be in a coma is:
    (1) Taste
    (2) Touch
    (3) Smell
    (4) Hearing

21. To best assist an agitated patient, the nurse should:
    (1) Focus on something other than the patient's agitation
    (2) Encourage the patient to share her feelings
    (3) Move her room next to the nurses' station
    (4) Keep the patient as active as possible

22. Mrs. Minetti, who is elderly, reminisces extensively and attempts to keep the nurse from leaving the room. The nurse's *most* therapeutic response would be:
    (1) Encouraging her to focus on the present and future
    (2) Limiting the amount of time she talks about the past
    (3) Suggesting that she reminisce with people her own age
    (4) Setting aside time to listen to the stories about her past

23. An elderly patient is incontinent. When changing his gown and linens, the nurse's *best* intervention would be to say:
    (1) "I am a nurse. This is part of my job."
    (2) "This doesn't bother me. It often happens."
    (3) "This occurs all the time. Try not to feel bad."
    (4) "I am Mrs. Lee. I will change your gown and linens."

24. Mr. Jackson has cancer and is receiving chemotherapy. He says to the nurse, "I just want to be well enough to enjoy the holidays." The nurse recognizes that according to Kübler-Ross he is in the stage of grieving known as:
    (1) Denial
    (2) Acceptance
    (3) Bargaining
    (4) Depression

25. Mrs. Levine is friendly, has many visitors, and appears happy. However, when her daughter visits, Mrs. Levine cries and complains of pain, and the daughter becomes upset. The nurse should:
    (1) Encourage the patient to change her behavior
    (2) Continue to observe this situation from a distance
    (3) Explore the situation with Mrs. Levine and her daughter
    (4) Tell the daughter that Mrs. Levine usually does not cry

26. Mrs. Geller has difficulty expressing herself verbally because of a stroke (aphasia). To increase Mrs. Geller's ability to communicate, the nurse should:
    (1) Talk to her, but not expect a response
    (2) Encourage her to embellish with gestures
    (3) Anticipate her needs to reduce frustration
    (4) Ask questions that require a yes or no response

27. Several times a day, every day, Mr. Grant asks when he will be getting his medications. He receives medication at the same time every day. The most therapeutic intervention would be to:
    (1) Tell him to go to the nurse when it is time for his pills
    (2) Encourage him to remember when he should take his pills
    (3) Inform him when he will be getting his next medications
    (4) Make a sign for his room indicating medication times

28. A patient is upset and rambles about an incident that occurred earlier in the week. The nurse should first:
    (1) Ask the patient what is wrong
    (2) Identify the patient's concern
    (3) Recognize the patient is confused
    (4) Refocus the patient to the present

29. Defense mechanisms can be classified as:
    (1) Relief behaviors
    (2) Conscious behaviors
    (3) Somatizing behaviors
    (4) Manipulative behaviors

30. A true statement about Kübler-Ross' theory on death and dying is that people:
    (1) Ultimately reach the stage of acceptance
    (2) Can move back and forth between the stages
    (3) Generally pass through the stages smoothly
    (4) Should move progressively forward through the stages

31. Mrs. Ramirez is admitted to the hospital. When her family leaves, she begins to cry. The probable etiology of the crying is:
    (1) Anger
    (2) Guilt
    (3) Denial
    (4) Anxiety

32. A dying patient says to the nurse, "All my life I was fairly religious, but I am still worried about what happens after death." The nurse's best response would be:
    (1) "The unknown is often very frightening."
    (2) "If you were religious, you know God is forgiving."
    (3) "People with after-death experiences say it is peaceful."
    (4) "You must feel good about being religious all your life."

Rationales

1. (1) This focuses on the nurse rather than the patient.
    * (2) This directly involves the patient and invites the patient to relive a past experience.
    (3) Same as #1.
    (4) This asks for an opinion, rather than a sharing of past experience.

2. * (1) Touch denotes caring; this statement is direct and supportive while not reinforcing denial.
    (2) Although this statement identifies feelings, it supports denial.
    (3) This is abandonment.
    (4) Although this may be done later, the patient needs immediate support.

3.   (1) This individualizes care and supports dignity and self-esteem.
     * (2) Usually eating is an independent activity of daily living; for an adult, assistance with meals may precipitate feelings of dependence and regression.
       (3) This is motivating and supports independence, self-esteem, and self-actualization.
       (4) This provides emotional support because it reduces fear of the unknown and involves the patient in care.

4.   (1) Patients with expressive aphasia often can communicate using nonverbal behaviors, a picture board, or written messages.
       (2) Words, whether they are spoken or written, are verbal communication.
     * (3) Touch is a form of nonverbal communication that sends a variety of messages depending on the person's culture, sex, age, past experiences, and present situation; touch also invades a person's personal space.
       (4) This is untrue; people from different cultures and people in subgroups within the same culture place different values on words.

5.   (1) This is inappropriate; it comes to a conclusion that may be inaccurate.
       (2) This is too direct; it may put the patient on the defensive and cut off communication.
       (3) Same as #2.
     * (4) This identifies the behavior and provides an opportunity for the patient to verbalize further.

6.   (1) This abandons the patient at a time when the nurse should be supportive.
       (2) This may eventually be done, but the patient needs immediate support.
       (3) This is false reassurance.
     * (4) This identifies feelings, focuses on the patient, and provides an opportunity for the patient to share feelings.

7.   (1) This is a command that may demean the patient; it challenges the patient and may precipitate more abusive behavior.
     * (2) This interrupts the behavior and protects the other patient; walking to the room uses excess energy and talking promotes verbalization of feelings and concerns.
       (3) This is judgmental; this implies the patient is not calm. An agitated patient has too much energy to sit quietly.
       (4) This is inappropriate because it challenges the patient and puts the patient on the defensive; this is a direct question that the patient may or may not be able to answer.

8.   (1) Patients who are angry strike out with verbal abuse or sarcasm; this patient's statement reflects feelings of sadness and isolation.
     * (2) Repeating the patient's statement allows the patient to focus on what was said, validates what was said, and encourages communication.
       (3) This may or may not be true and denies the patient's feelings.
       (4) Same as #3.

9.   (1) Denial is an unconscious defense mechanism; this patient consciously and voluntarily refuses to talk about the birthday.
       (2) This is an assumption; there are not enough data to come to this conclusion.
       (3) Same as #2.
     * (4) This is a conscious protective mechanism where a person actively puts anxiety-producing feelings or concerns out of the mind.

10. * (1) Pointing out the patient's behavior brings it to the attention of the patient and provides an opportunity to explore feelings.
     (2) The patient's behavior needs to be addressed more fully than would be possible with only continued observation.
     (3) This would be abandonment; sad, withdrawn patients need to know that they are accepted and that the nurse is available for support.
     (4) This denies the patient's feelings.

11. (1) This response uses reflective technique because it identifies a feeling. Also, this feeling was not expressed by the patient.
     (2) The patient's statement does not reflect feelings of sorrow or guilt.
     * (3) This restates the message using different words; paraphrasing focuses on content rather than the feeling or underlying emotional theme.
     (4) This is echolalia, not paraphrasing, because it uses the exact same words used by the patient.

12. (1) This is inappropriate; the patient is in the fourth stage of grieving, depression. During this stage people become quiet and withdrawn; the nurse should be quiet and available, not demonstrative.
     (2) This is inappropriate; cheerfulness denies the patient's feelings and cuts off communication.
     * (3) The patient is developing a full awareness of the impact of dying and is expressing sorrow; this stage of coping should be supported by the quiet presence of the nurse.
     (4) This would be a form of abandonment; the nurse must be present and accessible.

13. (1) This is future-oriented thinking and may be a form of bargaining for more time.
     * (2) When patients are depressed, they may feel a loss of control, alone, and withdrawn; when depressed, there is little physical energy, a lack of concern about the activities of daily living, and a decreased interest in physical appearance.
     (3) This behavior is associated with denial and bargaining.
     (4) This behavior reflects feelings of anger.

14. (1) This is inappropriate; the patient is unable to cope, is selecting the ultimate escape, and is not capable of meeting another person's needs. This response may also precipitate feelings such as guilt.
     (2) This denies the patient's feelings; the patient must focus on the negatives before exploring the positives.
     * (3) Open-ended statements identify feelings and invite further communication.
     (4) This is a judgmental response that may cut off communication; this is too direct, and the patient may not consciously know what is wrong.

15. (1) Shouting is demeaning and unnecessary; enunciating the words slowly and directly in front of the patient supports communication.
     (2) This is unrealistic. Communication is a two-way process; the patient is not having difficulty sending messages but rather is having difficulty receiving messages. This intervention is more appropriate for a patient with expressive aphasia.
     * (3) Communication can be promoted in a written, rather than a verbal, form; this reduces social isolation and promotes communication.
     (4) The patient is having difficulty with receiving, not sending, messages.

16. * (1) Touch is a simple form of communication that is easily understood even by confused, disoriented, or mentally incapacitated individuals.
    (2) This requires interpretation of symbols, which is a more complex form of communication than touch.
    (3) Same as #2.
    (4) Same as #2.

17. (1) This puts the focus on the nurse and cuts off communication.
    (2) This is inappropriate; opinions involve judgments that are based on feelings and values which may be different from the patient's.
    (3) While this might eventually be done, the patient's concerns and perceived alternatives should be explored first; also the patient may never want to talk about a particular concern with family members.
    * (4) This provides an opportunity for the patient to explore concerns and options without others influencing the decision making.

18. * (1) This recognizes the patient's behavior and provides an opportunity to verbalize feelings and concerns.
    (2) This is false reassurance.
    (3) This is inappropriate; this implies that the patient is out of control. This interferes with the patient's coping mechanisms and may not help the patient regain control.
    (4) This is false reassurance; crying may or may not help this patient.

19. (1) This is inappropriate because it denies the patient's feelings; the patient needs to focus on the future loss.
    (2) Same as #1.
    * (3) Depression is the fourth stage of dying according to Dr. Kübler-Ross; patients become withdrawn and noncommunicative when feeling a loss of control and recognizing future losses; the nurse should accept the behavior and be available if the patient wants to verbalize feelings.
    (4) It is never appropriate to offer advice; people must explore their alternatives and come to their own conclusions.

20. (1) Although all the senses are important, the ability to hear is the most important sense to an unconscious person.
    (2) Same as #1.
    (3) Same as #1.
    * (4) Hearing is the most important sense to an unconscious patient because it is believed it is the last sense that is lost; the senses receive stimuli from the environment and hearing keeps one in contact with others.

21. (1) All behavior has meaning; therefore, the agitation cannot be ignored.
    * (2) Agitation is a response to anxiety; the patient's feelings and concerns must be addressed to help relieve the anxiety and agitation.
    (3) Although this might be done, unless the cause of the agitation is identified and addressed, it will not decrease the agitation.
    (4) This could increase the agitation, particularly if the cause of the agitation is ignored.

22. (1) This is inappropriate; the developmental task of the elderly is to perform a life review.
    (2) Same as #1.

      (3) Patients should not be responsible for meeting each other's needs.

* (4) The nurse is responsible for assisting the patient to explore the past and deal with the developmental conflict of integrity versus despair.

23.   (1) This cuts off communication and puts the focus on the nurse rather than the patient; the patient also has the right to know who is providing care.

      (2) This generalizes, rather than individualizes, care; the focus should be on the patient. It also cuts off communication.

      (3) This is inappropriate; this implies the patient's behavior was bad.

* (4) This meets the patient's right to know who is providing care and what will be done; this is a nonjudgmental, respectful response that reduces fears of the unknown.

24.   (1) Denial is the first stage of disbelief, where the person avoids reality, is noncompliant, and uses emotional energy to deny the truth.

      (2) Acceptance is the fifth and final stage, where the person reminisces about the past, completes financial arrangements, and accepts death.

* (3) Bargaining is the third stage where the person is willing to do anything to change the prognosis, accepts new forms of therapies, and negotiates for more time.

      (4) Depression is the fourth stage where the person recognizes the future loss, withdraws from relationships to avoid feelings, and has feelings of loneliness.

25.   (1) This denies the patient's feelings and cuts off communication.

      (2) The nurse has a responsibility to intervene; the mother and daughter both have needs that must be met.

* (3) This provides an opportunity for both the mother and daughter to explore their feelings; all behavior has meaning and talking about the situation may provide insight.

      (4) This could further upset the daughter and may precipitate feelings such as guilt or anger.

26.   (1) Communication is a two-way process, and the patient should be involved; the patient should be encouraged to respond in some way.

* (2) Communication can be both verbal and nonverbal; this encourages communication.

      (3) Although this may be done occasionally, it does not increase the patient's ability to communicate.

      (4) Although this may be done occasionally, it does not increase the patient's ability to communicate; a yes or no response is too limited.

27.   (1) The patient probably would not be capable of this task; too challenging a task can be frustrating.

      (2) Same as #1.

      (3) Although this might be done, it is not the most therapeutic intervention because it addresses only the next dose.

* (4) This promotes independence and does not demean the patient; the patient can refer to the schedule when necessary.

28.   (1) This is too direct a statement; the patient may not be able to put into words what is wrong.

* (2) Active listening is necessary for data collection; once data are collected, the patient's feelings and concerns can be identified.

(3) When people are anxious, their conversation may ramble, but it does not necessarily mean that they are confused.

(4) This denies the patient's feelings; the patient will have to talk about the situation further to reduce anxiety.

29. * (1) Defense mechanisms are used to lower anxiety, manage stress, maintain the ego, and shelter self-esteem; while they can be productive or eventually detrimental, they do provide relief by releasing physical and emotional energy.

(2) Most defense mechanisms are utilized on an unconscious level, except for suppression which is used by the conscious mind.

(3) A somatizing behavior is identified when a patient experiences a psychological conflict as a physical symptom; physical symptoms distract the patient from the actual emotional distress as the patient internally manages the anxiety physiologically.

(4) Manipulative behaviors are not known as defense mechanisms but rather purposeful behaviors used to meet personal needs. Manipulative behaviors can be adaptive or maladaptive; they are maladaptive when they are the primary method used to meet needs, the needs of others are ignored, or others are dehumanized to meet the needs of the manipulator.

30. (1) This is untrue; some people never progress past denial; Kübler-Ross' theory of grieving is behaviorally oriented.

* (2) The stages are not concrete, and the patient's behavior changes as different levels of awareness and/or coping occur.

(3) Although this may be true for some people, it is not true for most individuals; the intensity and speed of progression depend on many factors such as extent of loss, level of growth and development, cultural and spiritual beliefs, sex roles, and relationships with significant others.

(4) This is untrue; patients tend to move back and forth among stages or may remain in one stage.

31. (1) Anger is usually expressed by acting-out aggressive behavior.

(2) Guilt is usually expressed by statements of sorrow and regret and behavior that attempts to make amends.

(3) Denial is a refusal to acknowledge facts that are consciously or unconsciously intolerable; a disregard for physical limitations or noncompliance with a medical regimen are examples of denial.

* (4) A change in a patient's emotional status, such as crying, usually reflects increased anxiety; crying releases physical and emotional tension and energy.

32. * (1) This uses reflective technique to identify the patient's feelings regarding fear of the unknown.

(2) This denies the patient's feelings and cuts off communication; also the patient's message did not indicate a need for forgiveness.

(3) This focuses on other peoples' experiences rather than the patient's feelings or concerns.

(4) This puts the emphasis on the wrong part of the message; it ignores the patient's concern about what happens after death.

PHYSICAL ASSESSMENT OF PATIENTS

This section encompasses questions related to various aspects of physical assessment. Questions focus on temperature, pulse, respirations, blood pressure, weight, level of consciousness, edema, and principles related to specimens and the collection of specimens. Additional questions focus on whether assessment data are subjective or objective in nature, whether sources are primary or secondary, the responsibilities of the nurse regarding data collected during assessment, the use of equipment to accurately collect data, assessments common to infection, the general adaptation syndrome, the inflammatory process, the sources of assessment data, and the use of common physical examination techniques.

Questions

1. A primary source assessing how a patient slept is the:
   (1) Primary nurse
   (2) Nurses' notes
   (3) Roommate
   (4) Patient

2. How long should the nurse wait to take an oral temperature after a patient has just had a cup of coffee?
   (1) 5 minutes
   (2) 7 minutes
   (3) 15 minutes
   (4) 30 minutes

3. The *best* source of information about a newly admitted alert patient with a fractured leg is the:
   (1) Emergency room nurse
   (2) Patient's family
   (3) Physician
   (4) Patient

4. The nurse should report which of the following signs and symptoms of respiratory distress to the physician?
   (1) Respiratory rate of 16 with a regular rhythm
   (2) Respiratory rate of 18 with shallow breathing
   (3) Respiratory rate of 20 with a regular rhythm
   (4) Respiratory rate of 26 with shallow breathing

5. When obtaining a radial pulse rate, the nurse understands that it reflects the function of the:
   (1) Arteries
   (2) Veins
   (3) Blood
   (4) Heart

6. An individual's body temperature would be at its lowest at:
   (1) 6 A.M.
   (2) 10 A.M.
   (3) 5 P.M.
   (4) 9 P.M.

7. When making rounds, the nurse finds a patient in bed with the eyes closed. The nurse should:
   (1) Suspect that the patient is feeling withdrawn
   (2) Return in 30 minutes to check on the patient
   (3) Collect more information about the patient
   (4) Allow the patient to continue sleeping

8. Which of the following is an example of objective data?
   (1) Pain
   (2) Fever
   (3) Nausea
   (4) Fatigue

9. Immediately after removing a glass theromometer from a patient's mouth, the nurse should first:
   (1) Rinse it with warm water
   (2) Wipe it dry with a tissue
   (3) Soak it in antiseptic solution
   (4) Wash it with soap and cool water

10. To assess if Mrs. Ramey is oriented, the nurse should:
    (1) Ask her to tell where she is and the time of day
    (2) Ascertain if she can follow simple directions
    (3) Inquire if she remembers the nurse's name
    (4) Determine if her eyes follow movement

11. When taking the pulse rate of an elderly patient, the nurse recognizes which of the following pulse ranges as normal?
    (1) 50 to 60 beats per minute
    (2) 80 to 90 beats per minute
    (3) 105 to 115 beats per minute
    (4) 120 to 130 beats per minute

12. Which of the following rectal temperatures is within the normal range?
    (1) 96.4°F
    (2) 97.6°F
    (3) 99.8°F
    (4) 101.2°F

13. Mr. Henry has a history of heart disease. After walking to the patient lounge, he sits in a chair, holds his hand against his chest, and complains of a severe upset stomach. The nurse should:
    (1) Walk him to his room
    (2) Take his vital signs
    (3) Administer an antacid
    (4) Listen to his complaints

14. How long should the nurse wait to take an oral temperature if the patient has just had a cold drink?
    (1) 3 minutes
    (2) 5 minutes
    (3) 15 minutes
    (4) 30 minutes

15. To assess for orthostatic hypotension, a patient's blood pressure should be measured:
    (1) Between meals
    (2) After standing
    (3) During activity
    (4) First thing in the morning

16. The general adaptation syndrome (GAS) is primarily controlled by the:
    (1) Endocrine system
    (2) Respiratory system
    (3) Integumentary system
    (4) Cardiovascular system

17. A patient's urine specific gravity is 1.035 indicating a need for:
    (1) Fluids
    (2) Protein
    (3) Glucose
    (4) Antibiotics

18. An example of subjective data is that the patient:
    (1) Appears jaundiced
    (2) Has a headache
    (3) Looks tired
    (4) Is crying

19. The diastolic blood pressure reflects which of the following physiological actions?
    (1) Contraction of the ventricles
    (2) Resting arterial pressure
    (3) Volume of cardiac output
    (4) Pulse pressure

20. When assessing a patient for an emotional response to stress, the patient should be monitored for:
    (1) Anorexia
    (2) Headaches
    (3) Irritability
    (4) Hypertension

21. When obtaining a pedal pulse, the nurse is assessing the function of the patient's:
    (1) Veins
    (2) Heart
    (3) Blood
    (4) Arteries

22. To ensure the most accurate results of a urine culture and sensitivity, the nurse should:
    (1) Obtain a double-voided specimen
    (2) Collect a midstream urine sample
    (3) Use the first voiding of the day
    (4) Utilize a 24-hour urine collection

23. Which of the following statements regarding blood pressure (BP) is true?
    (1) A BP differs 5 to 10 mm Hg between arms.
    (2) The second sound is more intense than the first.
    (3) A BP remains consistent regardless of the patient's position.
    (4) The arm must be kept below the apex of the heart to obtain an accurate BP.

24. When assessing for a systemic adaptation to an inflammatory response, the nurse should monitor the patient for:
    (1) Pain
    (2) Edema
    (3) Fever
    (4) Erythema

25. Which of the following physical examination techniques would elicit the most significant information concerning a patient's respiratory status?
    (1) Palpation
    (2) Percussion
    (3) Inspection
    (4) Auscultation

26. Which of the following BP readings would be considered the most hypertensive?
    (1) 90/70
    (2) 120/80

(3) 150/115
(4) 160/90

27. A concern that is common to the collection of specimens, regardless of their source, for culture and sensitivity tests is:
    (1) The specimen should be collected in the morning
    (2) Gloves, a gown, and a mask should be worn
    (3) Surgical asepsis must be maintained
    (4) Two specimens should be obtained

28. When assessing the pulse of an elderly woman, the nurse identifies a change from 88 to 56. The nurse should first:
    (1) Wait 15 minutes and retake the pulse
    (2) Ask the patient about her activity
    (3) Assess the other vital signs
    (4) Alert the charge nurse

29. When assessing cardiac function, the nurse recognizes which of the following as a principle of BP physiology?
    (1) A trough pressure occurs during systole.
    (2) The pulse pressure occurs during diastole.
    (3) A peak pressure occurs when the ventricles relax.
    (4) The blood pressure reaches a peak followed by a trough.

30. When obtaining a specimen from a wound for culture and sensitivity, the nurse should swab the wound at the:
    (1) Top
    (2) Edge
    (3) Bottom
    (4) Middle

31. The nurse recognizes that an inflammatory response has entered the second phase when the patient develops:
    (1) Pain
    (2) A fever
    (3) Erythema
    (4) An exudate

32. When assessing a patient for an initial response associated with the general adaptation syndrome (GAS), the nurse should monitor the patient for a:
    (1) Fluctuating blood pressure
    (2) Rising respiratory rate
    (3) Wavering mental acuity
    (4) Decreasing heart rate

33. When collecting a stool specimen for parasites, a consideration that is unique from other stool specimens is the need to:
    (1) Wear protective gloves
    (2) Obtain three successive daily specimens
    (3) Take feces from several areas of the bowel movement
    (4) Send the specimen to the laboratory while still warm

34. When assessing the results of a culture and sensitivity report, the sensitivity part of the test directly indicates the:
    (1) Type of microorganisms present
    (2) Virility of the organisms in the culture
    (3) Antibiotics that would be effective treatment
    (4) Extent of the patient's response to the pathogens

35. The nurse needs to recognize the patient's health beliefs because prior to giving care, the nurse must first:
    (1) Identify the patient's level of wellness
    (2) Understand the patient's frame of reference
    (3) Individualize the patient's nursing care plan
    (4) Teach the patient acceptable values related to health

Rationales

1. (1) This is a secondary source; the nurse may not be totally aware of how well the patient slept.
    (2) This is a secondary source that reflects history; the nurse who did the charting may not have been totally aware of how well the patient slept.
    (3) Patients should not be held responsible for other patients.
  * (4) The patient is the primary source and the only source able to provide subjective data concerning how she or he slept.
2. (1) This is too short a period of time for the mouth to recover from the hot fluid; the dilated vessels in the mouth and the warmth of the tissues from the hot fluid would cause an inaccurate elevation in the temperature reading.
    (2) Same as #1.
  * (3) It takes 15 minutes for the vessels in the mouth and the mucous membranes to recover from the hot fluid and for the mouth to return to the patient's core temperature.
    (4) This is unnecessary; this is too long a time period.
3. (1) This is a secondary source; when a patient is alert, the patient is the best source for current information.
    (2) Same as #1.
    (3) Same as #1.
  * (4) The patient is the center of the health team and is the primary source for current objective and subjective data.
4. (1) This is within the normal range of 12 to 20 breaths per minute; normal breathing is smooth and regular.
    (2) Normal breathing can be shallow if unlabored and within the acceptable rate of 12 to 20 breaths per minute.
    (3) Same as #1.
  * (4) Tachypnea, a respiratory rate above 24 breaths per minute, along with shallow breaths, indicate the body is compensating to meet oxygen needs.
5. (1) Elasticity and rigidity of the vessel walls and the quality and equality of pulses provide data about the status of the arteries.
    (2) A pulse is palpated in an artery, not a vein.
    (3) This is assessed through laboratory tests performed on blood specimens.
  * (4) The heart is a pulsatile pump that ejects blood into the arterial system with each ventricular contraction; the pulse is the vibration transmitted with each contraction.
6. * (1) A person's body temperature is at its lowest in the early morning; core temperatures vary with a predictable pattern over 24 hours (diurnal or circadian temperature variations) due to hormonal variations.
    (2) It is not at its lowest temperature at this time; body temperatures steadily rise as the day progresses.

       (3) Body temperatures peak between 4 and 7 P.M.

       (4) It is not at its lowest temperature at this time; the temperature is still falling from its peak.

7.   (1) This is an assumption based on insufficient data.

       (2) This is unsafe; more data needs to be collected at this time.

  * (3) More information must be collected to make a complete assessment and come to an accurate conclusion.

       (4) This is unsafe; this is an assumption based on insufficient data; a further assessment should be performed.

8.   (1) This is subjective; subjective data are a patient's perceptions, feelings sensations, or ideas.

  * (2) This is objective because it can be measured with a thermometer.

       (3) Same as #1.

       (4) Same as #1.

9.   (1) This would raise the mercury in the thermometer producing an inaccurate reading; this also could damage the thermometer.

  * (2) This removes mucus which may distort the level of the mercury or the numbers on the thermometer resulting in an inaccurate reading.

       (3) This is done after the reading has been taken and the thermometer has been washed in soap and water.

       (4) This is done after the reading has been taken.

10. * (1) Questions related to time, place, in addition to person (oriented times 3) are essential when assessing a patient's level of orientation.

       (2) This is inaccurate; this can be done by confused, disoriented patients.

       (3) This assesses recent memory, not orientation.

       (4) Same as #2.

11.   (1) This is below the normal range of a pulse rate in an elderly patient.

  * (2) The normal heart rate in an adult is between 60 and 100 beats per minute.

       (3) This is too high for a heart rate taken at rest; in the elderly a decreased contractile strength of the myocardium causes the heart rate to increase more than usual during exercise.

       (4) This is too high for a heart rate taken at rest.

12.   (1) This is outside the normal range for a rectal temperature; it is too low.

       (2) Same as #1.

  * (3) This is within the normal range of 98.6 to 100.6°F for a rectal temperature.

       (4) This would be a fever.

13.   (1) This is unsafe; if the problem is cardiac, rather than gastric, walking will increase the demands on the heart.

  * (2) A further assessment is necessary; vital signs reflect the cardiopulmonary status of the patient.

       (3) The nurse needs more information before concluding the problem is gastritis; antacids require a physician's order.

       (4) Although this would be done, it is most important that the nurse collect objective data about the patient's cardiopulmonary status.

14.   (1) This is too short a time period; the mucous membranes will be cool and the vessels in the mouth will be constricted resulting in an inaccurate reduction in temperature.

       (2) Same as #1.

* (3) It takes 15 minutes for the mucous membranes and vessels in the mouth to recover from the cold fluid and return to the patient's core temperature.

(4) This is unnecessary; this is too long a period of time.

15.   (1) This is untrue; this is unrelated to positional changes.

* (2) Blood pressures taken before and after standing reflect the effectiveness of the autonomic vasoconstriction that occurs in the lower half of the body when a patient moves from a horizontal to a vertical position; vasoconstriction prevents pooling of blood and effectively maintains the blood pressure.

(3) This is done during a stress test.

(4) This is a blood pressure at rest.

16. * (1) The general adaptation syndrome (GAS) primarily involves the endocrine system and autonomic nervous system; the antidiuretic hormone (ADH), adrenocorticotropic hormone (ACTH), cortisol, aldosterone, epinephrine, and norepinephrine are all involved with the fight-or-flight response.

(2) This system will be stimulated by the hormone epinephrine.

(3) The autonomic nervous system affects the integumentary system.

(4) This system will be stimulated by the hormones epinephrine and norepinephrine.

17. * (1) Specific gravity indicates the degree of concentration of dissolved substances in the urine; the normal specific gravity is 1.010 to 1.025; the higher the specific gravity, the more concentrated the urine. Concentrated urine indicates dehydration; when a patient is dehydrated, fluids are indicated.

(2) Specific gravity is not designed to test for nitrogen balance; a negative nitrogen balance indicates the need for increased protein intake. Excessive protein in the urine indicates clinical conditions such as nephritis, cardiac failure, mercury poisoning, or hematuria. However, it does not indicate the need for increased fluid intake.

(3) Specific gravity is not designed to test the level of glucose in the urine; glucose in the urine is measured by a Clinitest tablet, Keto-Diastix, or Multistix reagent strip. Glucose in the urine indicates conditions such as diabetes mellitus, pituitary disorders, or increased intracranial pressure.

(4) Specific gravity is not designed to test for the presence of an infection; an increased white blood cell count or a positive culture and sensitivity indicated the presence of infection and the need for antibiotics.

18.   (1) This is objective data; objective data require the use of a sense to collect the data. Jaundice is a human response that is measured using the sense of vision and the assessment technique of inspection.

* (2) Subjective data are data that can be described or verified only by the patient; a patient's descriptions of pain, concerns, feelings, or sensations are additional examples of subjective data.

(3) This is a conclusion.

(4) Same as #1.

19.   (1) This is reflected by the systolic pressure.

* (2) Diastole is the period when the ventricles are relaxed and reflects the pressure in the arteries when the heart is at rest.

(3) The volume of cardiac output is computed by multiplying the stroke volume by the number of heartbeats per minute.

(4) This is the difference between the systolic and diastolic pressures.

20.   (1) This is a physiological response to stress.
        (2) Same as #1.
    *   (3) This is a behavioral-emotional response; the body is utilizing physical and emotional energy to reduce stress.
        (4) Same as #1.

21.   (1) Veins do not have a pulse.
        (2) A radial, carotid, or apical pulse more readily assesses heart function.
        (3) Laboratory tests assess blood and its components.
    *   (4) The presence, absence, or quality of a pedal pulse reflects the patency of the dorsalis pedis artery; peripheral pulses should be present, equal, and symmetrical.

22.   (1) A double-voided specimen is taken for the measurement of glucose and ketones in the urine; stagnant urine from the bladder does not reflect a current level of glucose and ketones in the urine being produced at the time of the voiding.
    *   (2) This method obtains a urine specimen that is relatively free of microorganisms from the urethra; after perineal care the patient begins to void discarding the initial stream and collecting a specimen during the midportion of the stream. Perineal care and the initial stream clear the urethra of microorganisms providing for a specimen with the least amount of contamination.
        (3) Specimens collected from the first voiding of the morning should be avoided; stagnant urine does not reflect urine that is recently filtered by the urinary system. A first voiding does not allow for the clearing of the urethra of growing microorganisms as in the midstream collection method.
        (4) This is unnecessary; 24 hours of urine is needed for special tests such as the measurement of levels of adrenocortical steroids, hormones, and creatinine clearance tests, not for a urine culture and sensitivity.

23. * (1) Because of variations in structure and distance, there might be 5 to 10 mm Hg difference between arms; the arm with the higher blood pressure should be used for subsequent assessments.
        (2) The opposite is true.
        (3) This is untrue; the blood pressure is higher when the arm is below heart level and lower when the arm is above heart level.
        (4) This would result in an abnormally lower blood pressure; the arm should be at the apex of the heart.

24.   (1) This is a local adaptation to stimulation of nerve endings; it is a localized response of the central nervous system to the stimulus of pain.
        (2) This is a local adaptation resulting from local vasodilation and increased vessel permeability.
    *   (3) The inflammatory response is stimulated by trauma or infection which increase the basal metabolic rate; with infection fever results from the affect of pyrogens on the temperature-regulating center in the hypothalamus.
        (4) This is a local adaptation resulting from increased circulation and local vasodilation in the involved area.

25. (1) Although the chest wall is palpated for bulges, tenderness, respiratory excursion, and vocal fremitus which provide valuable information, auscultation of breath sounds provides the most significant information concerning a patient's respiratory status.

(2) Although percussion of the thorax determines whether underlying tissue is filled with air, liquid, or solid material and identifies the boundaries of the lung, auscultation of breath sounds provides the most significant information concerning a patient's respiratory status.

(3) Although inspection assesses the pattern of respirations, condition of the skin, and shape and symmetry of the thorax, auscultation of breath sounds provides the most significant information concerning a patient's respiratory status.

* (4) Auscultation of the chest includes assessment of breath sounds (normal, diminished, absent); adventitious breath sounds (rales or crackles, rhonchi, wheeze, friction rub); and vocal resonance (bronchophony, whispered pectoriloquy, egophony). This information is the most significant for assessing the patient's respiratory status.

26. (1) This is hypotensive.

(2) This is within the normal range for blood pressure; the normal range for the systolic pressure is 100 to 140, and the diastolic pressure is 60 to 90.

* (3) A blood pressure with a higher diastolic pressure is more hypertensive than a blood pressure with a higher systolic pressure but lower diastolic pressure. The diastolic pressure is the pressure exerted against the arterial walls when the ventricles are at rest; the higher the diastolic, the more dangerous the situation.

(4) While this systolic reading is high and needs to be reported to the physician, a blood pressure with a higher diastolic is more dangerous.

27. (1) The time of day is irrelevant for the collection of most specimens for culture and sensitivity.

(2) Gloves may be worn when collecting specimens to protect the nurse, not to maintain sterility of the specimen; gowns and masks are generally unnecessary unless splashing of body fluids is likely.

* (3) The results of a culture and sensitivity are faulty and erroneous if the collection container is not kept sterile; a contaminated specimen container introduces extraneous microorganisms that falsify and misrepresent results. Surgical asepsis (sterile technique) must be maintained.

(4) Generally if a specimen is collected using proper technique, one specimen is sufficient for testing for culture and sensitivity. However, blood cultures for a disease such as endocarditis may require several specimens over a 24- to 48-hour period.

28. (1) This is unsafe; when there is an alteration in one vital sign, the other vital signs should immediately be taken.

(2) Activity would increase, not decrease, the heart rate.

* (3) Corroborative data should be obtained; the vital signs reflect cardiopulmonary functioning. When there is an alteration in one vital sign, there is usually a change in another.

(4) This might be necessary after taking the other vital signs.

29. (1) Peak pressures occur during systole.

(2) Pulse pressure is the difference between the systolic and diastolic pressure.

(3) Peak pressures occur when the ventricles contract.

* (4) Peak pressures occur when the ventricles contract, and trough pressures occur when the ventricles relax; these occur with each contraction and relaxation of the heart.

30. (1) Specimens collected from this area could be contaminated from microorganisms from the skin, misrepresenting results.

(2) Same as #1.

(3) Same as #1.

* (4) Swabbing from the center of a wound provides for a specimen that is least likely to be contaminated by microorganisms from the skin; it also provides for a specimen that generally contains the most representative properties of the exudate.

31. (1) Pain occurs during the first phase in response to the release of histamine at the injury site; histamine promotes vessel permeability, which increases edema causing pressure on nerve endings.

(2) Fever is a systemic adaptation and is not indicative of phase 2 of the inflammatory response.

(3) During the first phase histamine is released which results in increased blood flow to the area; dilation of capillaries causes the area to be flooded with blood, which makes the area appear red and warm to the touch.

* (4) Phase 2 is characterized by the formation of an exudate; it consists of a combination of cells and fluids produced at the injury site.

32. (1) Because of the effects of the sympathetic nervous system, the blood pressure will rise, not fluctuate.

* (2) The sympathetic nervous system response results in bronchial dilation and an increased respiratory rate; this increases the amount of oxygen available for the elevated basal metabolic rate associated with the general adaptation syndrome (GAS).

(3) Because of the sympathetic nervous system response, the individual's mental ability is alert and constant in preparation for the "fight"; the mental acuity does not waver.

(4) Because of the effects of the sympathetic nervous system, the heart rate increases, not decreases.

33. (1) Gloves should always be worn when dealing with body secretions or excretions.

(2) Three separate samples from stool are collected on consecutive days to screen for occult blood, not for parasites.

(3) This is unnecessary; a 1-inch portion of stool provides an adequate sample for testing for parasites.

* (4) Stool specimens for ova and parasites should be sent to the laboratory while still warm; stool that is allowed to cool can alter the accuracy of the laboratory results.

34. (1) Examination of a specimen under a microscope identifies the microorganisms present.

(2) The ability to produce disease (virulence) is not determined by the sensitivity portion of a culture and sensitivity; virulence is determined by statistical data concerning morbidity and mortality associated with the microorganism.

* (3) Areas of lack of growth of microorganisms surrounding an antibiotic on a culture medium indicate that the microorganism is sensitive to the antibiotic and the antibiotic is capable of destroying the microorganism.
  (4) The sensitivity part of a culture and sensitivity test refer to the ability of an antibiotic to destroy a microorganism, not an individual's susceptibility to or extent of response to the microorganism.

35.   (1) This occurs after the nurse understands the variables influencing the patient's attitudes, beliefs, and practices.
* (2) Attitudes and beliefs influence health practices and how one perceives self-health; the nurse must always "begin care where the patient is at."
  (3) Same as #1.
  (4) This is judgmental; people perceive their values as acceptable.

MEETING PATIENTS' HEALTH AND SAFETY NEEDS

This section encompasses questions related to maintaining patients' physical health and safety. A particular emphasis is placed on the concepts of medical asepsis; the use of restraints; bed making; issues associated with smoking; prevention of injury; fire safety; the use of devices to support safety; interventions to protect a patient having a seizure; use of the call bell; interventions and use of devices to prevent falls; electrical safety; safety related to oxygen use; principles related to various types of isolation; and post-mortem care.

Questions

1. When applying a wrist restraint, what should the nurse do to avoid injury to the patient?
   (1) Pad the wrist with sheepskin
   (2) Secure the strap to the bed rail
   (3) Release the restraint every 3 hours
   (4) Tie the strap loosely around the wrist

2. The nurse should encourage the patient to wash the hands before and after voiding. Washing the hands prior to voiding can be evaluated as effective when the patient is:
   (1) Able to void
   (2) In fluid balance
   (3) Free from infection
   (4) Emotionally comfortable

3. When soiled linen is removed from a bed, it should be placed:
   (1) In a linen hamper
   (2) On the overbed table
   (3) Into the linen chute
   (4) On a chair

4. If a patient becomes more confused after a restraint has been applied, the nurse should:
   (1) Administer the ordered sedative
   (2) Encourage the patient to relax
   (3) Remove the restraint
   (4) Reorient the patient

5. A patient must be restrained while out of bed in a chair. To provide for this patient's safety, the nurse should:
   (1) Avoid the use of a wheelchair
   (2) Place the patient near the door
   (3) Reposition the patient every 3 hours
   (4) Position a call bell next to the patient

6. To prevent accidents because of smoking in facilities that are not "smoke free," the nurse should:
   (1) Encourage patients not to smoke
   (2) Inform patients that they cannot smoke
   (3) Instruct patients to smoke in smoking areas
   (4) Keep the patient's cigarettes at the nurses' station

7. The *main* reason for accidents in hospitals is:
   (1) Patients sneak cigarettes
   (2) Equipment breaks unexpectedly
   (3) People do not recognize hazards
   (4) Safety precautions take extra time

8. Restraints are mainly used to:
   (1) Immobilize patients
   (2) Reduce agitation
   (3) Limit movement
   (4) Prevent injury

9. Bacteria rapidly multiply in environments that are:
   (1) Hot
   (2) Warm
   (3) Cool
   (4) Cold

10. Linens that are still clean are often reused by the same patient. The article of linen that is *least* likely to be reused is the:
    (1) Top sheet
    (2) Bedspread
    (3) Pillowcase
    (4) Cotton blanket

11. Mrs. Glazer is sitting in a wheelchair and begins to have a seizure. The nurse should:
    (1) Wheel her immediately to her room for privacy
    (2) Return her to her bed to provide a soft surface
    (3) Move her to the floor to prevent injury
    (4) Secure her in the wheelchair so she does not fall

12. A patient on contact isolation needs a blood pressure taken every shift. To keep the sphygmomanometer from spreading microorganisms, the most practical intervention by the nurse would be to:
    (1) Place it in a protective bag
    (2) Keep it in the patient's room
    (3) Store it in the dirty utility room
    (4) Wipe it down with a germicidal solution

13. Disoriented, confused patients who are restrained often struggle against restraints primarily because they are:
    (1) Unable to understand what is occurring
    (2) Trying to manipulate the staff
    (3) Responding to the discomfort
    (4) Attempting to gain control

14. After a patient vomits, the nurse should:
    (1) Pour the vomitus down the sink in the dirty utility room
    (2) Contain vomitus in the medical waste container
    (3) Discard the vomitus in the toilet and flush
    (4) Save a specimen for the physician

15. In institutions that are not smoke free, the nurse can BEST prevent accidents associated with smoking by:
    (1) Supervising patients when they smoke
    (2) Taking away the cigarettes of patients who smoke
    (3) Encouraging patients to smoke in their own rooms
    (4) Asking family members not to bring cigarettes for patients

16. Mr. Brown dies. As part of postmortem care, the nurse should:
    (1) Slightly raise the head of the bed
    (2) Firmly tie the wrists together
    (3) Carefully remove the dentures
    (4) Gently close the eyes

17. The nurse should remove a dirty sheet from an unoccupied bed by:
    (1) Pushing it together
    (2) Folding up the sheet
    (3) Rolling it into itself
    (4) Fan-folding it to the side

18. While transporting a fire extinguisher to a fire scene on a level of the building different from the one on which the nurse is working, the nurse should:
    (1) Use the stairs
    (2) Pull the safety pin
    (3) Run as quickly as possible
    (4) Keep it from touching the floor

19. The first thing the staff nurse should review with a newly admitted patient is the:
    (1) Use of the call bell
    (2) Name of the charge nurse
    (3) Daily routine on the unit
    (4) Potential date of discharge

20. To prevent disorientation at night in the minimally confused patient, the most effective intervention would be to:
    (1) Describe the environment prior to sleep
    (2) Turn on a small light in the room
    (3) Check on the patient regularly
    (4) Place a call bell in the bed

21. While assisting Mrs. Green with ambulation, she becomes weak and her knees begin to buckle. The nurse should:
    (1) Support her to keep her from falling
    (2) Lower her to the floor gently
    (3) Walk her to the closest chair
    (4) Call for extra help quickly

22. The most effective method to prevent confused patients from falling out of bed is the:
    (1) Use of vest restraints
    (2) Raising of bedside rails
    (3) Administration of sedatives
    (4) Lowering the height of the bed

23. When changing the bed linens, the nurse decides to reuse the blanket because it is still clean. The nurse should:
    (1) Store it on the floor of the patient's closet
    (2) Reconsider and replace it with a new blanket
    (3) Fan-fold it to the foot of the patient's bed
    (4) Place it on the windowsill out of the way

24. When the nurse finds that the electrical cord on a patient's radio is frayed near the plug, the nurse should:
    (1) Remove it and send it home with a family member
    (2) Wrap the frayed area with nonconductive tape
    (3) Unplug it and put it in the patient's closet
    (4) Report it to the supervisor

25. A patient with a vest restraint should have the restraint released and activity provided every:
    (1) 30 minutes
    (2) hour
    (3) 2 hours
    (4) 4 hours

26. Which of the following would have the greatest impact on limiting the spread of microorganisms?
    (1) Disposable equipment
    (2) Double-bagging
    (3) Handwashing
    (4) Gloves

27. An unacceptable practice related to the application of wrist restraints is:
    (1) Using a double knot to secure the straps
    (2) Securing the ties to the base of the bed
    (3) Allowing the fingers free movement
    (4) Padding the wrists with sheepskin

28. Mr. Crowley chews tobacco and likes to spit his tobacco juice on the floor. What should the nurse do *first?*
    (1) Encourage him to use chewing gum instead
    (2) Teach him to dispose of his saliva safely
    (3) Keep the chewing tobacco at the nurses' station
    (4) Inform him that he should chew the tobacco in his room

29. When planning nursing interventions to prevent falls in the elderly, the nurse recognizes that the frequency of falls increase:
    (1) At night
    (2) After meals
    (3) During visiting hours
    (4) When getting up in the morning

30. To provide for safety when administering oxygen, it is most important that the nurse first recognize that oxygen:
    (1) Must have its flow rate adjusted
    (2) Is drying to the nasal mucosa
    (3) Should be humidified
    (4) Supports combustion

31. Which of the following actions is specific to caring for a patient on respiratory isolation?
    (1) Keeping the patient's door closed
    (2) Donning a gown when administering medications

(3) Wearing disposable gloves when delivering a meal
(4) Instructing the patient to wear a mask when receiving care

Rationales

1. * (1) This is appropriate; the wrist has several bony prominences and little muscle or adipose tissue to protect this area from pressure and skin breakdown.
   (2) This is unsafe; an extremity can be injured if the bed rail is lowered while the strap is still tied to the rail. Also the side rail is not stationary. Always tie a restraint strap to the frame under the bed.
   (3) Restraints are required to be released a minimum of every 2 hours and whenever necessary; this is a basic standard of practice.
   (4) This is unsafe; it should be tied snugly yet loosely enough so as not to impede circulation or cause discomfort.

2. (1) Handwashing is done to remove microorganisms, not to induce voiding.
   (2) Handwashing is related to reducing microorganisms not fluid balance.
   * (3) Handwashing prevents the patient from becoming contaminated by soiled hands.
   (4) Handwashing is related to meeting physical needs, not emotional needs.

3. * (1) This is acceptable practice; this is a safe way to contain microorganisms.
   (2) This is unsafe; the overbed table is considered a clean surface and should not be used to hold soiled linen. This action will contaminate the overbed table.
   (3) This is unsafe; soiled linen should be bagged before it is deposited in a linen chute.
   (4) This is unsafe; a chair is considered a clean surface and should not us used to hold soiled linen. This action will contaminate the chair.

4. (1) A sedative is a chemical restraint. Use of two kinds of restraints is undesirable.
   (2) This denies the patient's feelings and does not address the confusion.
   (3) This would be unsafe.
   * (4) Reorienting the patient and reinforcing explanations regarding the purpose of the restraint contribute to understanding and compliance.

5. (1) A patient can be safely restrained in a wheelchair.
   (2) This would be too far from the call bell.
   (3) This should be done every 2 hours.
   * (4) A patient who is restrained should be in the direct view of the nurse or have a call bell to summon help if needed.

6. (1) Although many facilities are smoke free, some permit smoking if safely done in designated areas; these patients have a right to smoke.
   (2) Same as #1.
   * (3) Education increases understanding and compliance with safety rules. This limits smoking to supervised areas.
   (4) Patients have a right to keep their cigarettes as long as they adhere to the safety regulations.

7. (1) Supervision helps to minimize this risk, and statistics do not support this as the main reason for hospital accidents.
   (2) Equipment is usually monitored for preventive maintenance; equipment generally shows wear and tear before it breaks.

* (3) Patients can be cognitively impaired, deny their physical impairments, or have limited perception, all of which can impede their ability to recognize hazards.

(4) This is not true; it often takes the same amount of time to do something correctly that it takes to do it incorrectly.

8. (1) Restraints should be snug yet loose enough for some movement; immobilization is not the purpose of restraints.

(2) Restraints can increase agitation; if used when a patient is severely agitated, they can cause injury.

(3) The purpose of restraints is to prevent injury, not limit movement.

* (4) This is the primary reason for the use of restraints; they are used as a last resort to protect the patient from self-injury or from hurting others.

9. (1) Hot temperatures are used to destroy bacteria (e.g., sterilization).

* (2) Bacteria grows most rapidly in dark, warm, and moist environments.

(3) Bacteria grows best in temperature close to normal body temperature (98.6°F), not cool or cold environments.

(4) Same as #3.

10. (1) This is often used again if it is still clean.

(2) Same as #1.

* (3) This comes in contact with the hair; exudate from the eyes, mucus from the nose, and saliva from the mouth; it is easily soiled and usually needs to be replaced more often than other linens.

(4) Same as #1.

11. (1) Physical safety is the priority, not the need for privacy.

(2) Keeping the patient in the wheelchair while transporting her to her room could cause muscle strain, bones to fracture, or other injury; this should be done once the seizure is over.

* (3) This is the safest action; it provides for free movement on a supported surface.

(4) This could cause serious injury; moving the patient to the floor is the safest action.

12. (1) It must be taken out of the bag when used, thereby resulting in contamination.

* (2) This is the most practical; when isolation is discontinued, all equipment can be terminally disinfected.

(3) It is contaminated and needs to be disinfected before removal from the patient's room.

(4) This is safe but time-consuming; it is more practical to leave frequently used equipment in an isolation room.

13. * (1) This is true; disoriented and confused patients do not have the cognitive ability to always understand what is happening to them.

(2) A patient usually struggles against a restraint to get free, not to manipulate staff.

(3) A restraint should not cause discomfort if it is correctly applied and checked frequently.

(4) Confused, disoriented patients who are restrained may become agitated and respond in a reflexlike way; attempts to gain control require problem solving, which confused disoriented patients usually are unable to perform.

14. (1) It is unnecessary to remove vomitus from the room; vomitus should not be poured down a sink but rather into a toilet.

(2) This is unnecessary if the vomitus can be flushed down a toilet.

* (3) This is the safest and most practical action when disposing of vomitus; it dilutes, contains, and removes the vomitus.
  (4) This is usually unnecessary; while a physician may request that vomitus be assessed, it is rarely saved or sent for laboratory analysis.

15. * (1) If a facility allows smoking, supervision provides for patient safety because the nurse can intervene if the situation becomes unsafe.
   (2) In some facilities patients have a right to smoke if it is safely done in designated areas; the nurse should teach, rather than punish, the patient.
   (3) This is unsafe; smoking patients should be supervised.
   (4) This does not ensure patient safety; only supervised smoking protects the patient.

16. (1) A position of normal alignment is preferred; once rigor mortis sets in, it is difficult to reposition the body.
   (2) Firmly tying the wrists can cause permanent marks; wrists should be well padded and securely, yet loosely, tied so as not to cause permanent marks.
   (3) Dentures should remain in the mouth to maintain facial structure and minimize facial distortion.
  * (4) The eyelids should be gently closed to avoid injury; once rigor mortis sets in, it is difficult to reposition the eyelids.

17. (1) This would not secure loose ends; debris could fall on the floor.
   (2) Same as #1.
  * (3) This secures loose ends and keeps debris contained within the center of the sheet as it is rolled into itself.
   (4) Fan-folding is a method used to neatly stack a sheet on one side of a bed for ease in passing it under or over a patient; it is not a method used to remove a sheet in an effort to contain debris.

18. * (1) This is safe; elevators must be avoided because they could break down and trap a person.
   (2) The safety pin is pulled only when the extinguisher is going to be used, not when *en route* to a fire.
   (3) Running should be avoided; it can cause injury and panic.
   (4) Often extinguishers are dragged along the floor *en route* to a fire because they are heavy; this is acceptable practice.

19. * (1) This meets basic safety and security needs; the patient must know how to signal for help.
   (2) Although this is important and should be done, safety needs come first.
   (3) Same as #2.
   (4) This is the physician's responsibility.

20. (1) The patient may not remember the description of the environment upon awakening and could become disoriented in the dark.
  * (2) This would provide enough light for visual cues that would help prevent or minimize disorientation upon awakening at night.
   (3) While this is something the nurse should do to provide for patient safety, turning on a small light would be most effective in minimizing disorientation.
   (4) The patient has to be oriented enough to be aware of the presence of the call bell before it can be used; a small light would enable the patient to see the room and call bell.

21.   (1) This could injure the nurse and cause both the nurse and the patient to fall.
    * (2) This is the safest action; guiding the patient to the floor helps to break the fall and minimize injury.
       (3) The patient is already falling; this is not an option.
       (4) By the time help arrives, the patient may already be on the floor; calling out can scare the patient and others.

22. * (1) Of all the options offered, the vest restraint is the method that provides the most security to prevent a fall.
       (2) The patient can still climb over the rail and fall.
       (3) Sedation should not be used as a restraint.
       (4) While this might be done, it will not prevent a fall.

23.   (1) Items should never be stored on the floor of any area because they will become contaminated by microorganisms on the floor.
       (2) This is unnecessary; linen that is still clean can be reused for the same patient.
    * (3) This is a safe and practical way to store a blanket; a fan-folded blanket can be easily opened over the patient.
       (4) Used linen should never be placed on the windowsill; the blanket is considered contaminated.

24. * (1) This is the safest option; this option removes it from use.
       (2) This is unsafe; it should be repaired by a trained person.
       (3) This is unsafe; it can be taken out and used again.
       (4) This is unnecessary; it should be removed from use.

25.   (1) Circulation should be checked every 30 minutes; a restraint is released every 2 hours and exercise or activity provided.
       (2) This is unnecessary; a restraint is released every 2 hours.
    * (3) A restraint should be released every 2 hours, the area moved through range of motion, and the skin massaged with lotion.
       (4) This is too long; pressure can cause skin breakdown due to ischemia, and immobility can cause contractures.

26.   (1) While this helps reduce the spread of microorganisms, it still needs to be safely handled once used; handwashing is the most effective measure to reduce the spread of microorganisms.
       (2) This only is used to dispose of infectious waste; while it limits the spread of infection, handwashing is the most effective measure to reduce the spread of microorganisms.
    * (3) Handwashing is the most effective measure to reduce the spread of infection because it removes microorganisms from the hands.
       (4) Gloves protect the nurse; however, even when gloves are used, hands must be washed before and after use to prevent the spread of infection.

27. * (1) This is unsafe; a double knot prevents easy release in the event of an emergency.
       (2) This is safe; restraint straps should be tied to an immoveable underpart of the bed. This prevents injury when side rails are lowered; straps are also out of reach of the patient.
       (3) This is safe; the wrists, not the fingers, are restrained.
       (4) This is safe; the wrist has several bony prominences and little muscle or adipose tissue to protect this area from pressure and skin breakdown.

28.   (1) The patient has a right to chew tobacco as long as acceptable infection control guidelines are followed.
   * (2) This action provides information needed to meet acceptable expectations regarding the disposal of tobacco juice and saliva; if infection control principles are followed, the patient can chew tobacco.
     (3) This denies the right to chew tobacco and does not change the unsafe behavior; an effort must be made to educate the patient about safe disposal of tobacco juice and saliva.
     (4) This does not address the problem; the patient must be taught infection control principles because the patient may continue to spit tobacco juice on the floor.

29. * (1) Because of a dark, unfamiliar environment at night, elderly patients may become confused and disoriented which contributes to the occurrence of falls.
     (2) This is generally unrelated to falls.
     (3) Same as #2.
     (4) The risk of falls upon awakening is not as high as it is at night when the lights are dim or off; the light of day and the use of lights promote orientation.

30.   (1) Although this is true, safety is the priority.
     (2) Same as #1.
     (3) Same as #1.
   * (4) Although oxygen by itself will not burn or explode, it facilitates combustion; the greater the concentration of oxygen, the more rapidly fires start and burn.

31. * (1) Keeping the door closed prevents the spread of droplets in the air which may contain infectious microorganisms.
     (2) When administering medications to a patient on respiratory isolation, the nurse must wear a mask, not a gown; a mask is worn to protect the nurse from infectious droplets that may be in the air.
     (3) When delivering a meal tray to a patient on respiratory isolation, the nurse must wear a mask, not gloves.
     (4) The nurse wears the mask for self-protection, not the patient.

MEETING PATIENTS' HYGIENE AND COMFORT NEEDS

This section encompasses questions related to meeting patients' hygiene and comfort needs. Questions focus on theories of pain; assessment of pain; pain relief measures; rest and sleep; the backrub; bed making; the use of heat and cold; principles associated with bed baths; perineal care for male and female patients; and care of the eyes, hair, feet, and mouth.

Questions

1. Mr. Johnson has a high temperature, is diaphoretic, and did not sleep well during the night. When planning for Mr. Johnson's hygiene needs, the nurse should:
   (1) Give a complete bath
   (2) Do a partial bed bath
   (3) Delay the bath until later
   (4) Provide just perineal care

2. To support dignity when providing oral hygiene for a patient with dentures, the nurse should:
   (1) Provide a denture cup for the patient
   (2) Pull the curtain around the patient's bed
   (3) Support the patient in a high-Fowler's position
   (4) Resist looking at the patient while the dentures are out

3. When giving a patient a bed bath, the water temperature should be:
   (1) 80 to 90°F
   (2) 95 to 105°F
   (3) 110 to 115°F
   (4) 120 to 130°F

4. When administering perineal care, the nurse can *best* provide for emotional comfort by:
   (1) Placing the patient in the supine position
   (2) Pulling the curtain around the bed
   (3) Using warm water for washing
   (4) Calling the patient by name

5. When providing a partial bed bath, the nurse should:
   (1) Help the patient to wash the face, hands, underarms, back, and perineal area
   (2) Direct the patient to wash as much as possible and assist with the rest
   (3) Instruct the patient to wash the face, hands, and perineal area
   (4) Assist the patient to wash just one part of the body at at time

6. When the physician orders that a patient be kept NPO, the *most* important action by the nurse should be to:
   (1) Allow the patient to sip clear fluids with medication
   (2) Give the patient mouth care every 4 hours
   (3) Permit the patient to suck on ice chips
   (4) Measure the patient's intake and output

7. While administering a bed bath, the main reason the nurse rinses the patient after applying soap and water is to:
   (1) Increase circulation
   (2) Promote rest and comfort
   (3) Minimize decubitus ulcers
   (4) Remove residue and debris

8. When planning care for a patient with offensive mouth odor, the most effective intervention would be to encourage:
   (1) Eating foods that do not generate odors
   (2) Brushing the teeth and tongue after meals
   (3) Rinsing the mouth with mouthwash every shift
   (4) Cleaning the mouth with peroxide and baking soda

9. Which of the following would be least effective in preventing hair from tangling and matting?
   (1) Using conditioners after shampooing
   (2) Washing the hair with shampoo
   (3) Placing the hair in braids
   (4) Brushing the hair daily

10. To prevent decubitus ulcers, the bottom sheet should be:
    (1) Covered by a draw sheet
    (2) Kept free of wrinkles
    (3) Made with a toe pleat
    (4) Changed each day

11. Which of the following is within the correct range for the temperature of bath water?
    (1) 98.6°F
    (2) 105°F
    (3) 109°F
    (4) 113°F

12. Prior to discharge, an elderly patient complains of having dry, itchy skin. To limit these problems, the nurse should teach the patient to apply a lubricating lotion and:
    (1) Avoid the sun
    (2) Bathe every day
    (3) Wear short-sleeve shirts
    (4) Rub the itchy areas with a soft towel

13. What should the nurse do when a patient has tangled and matted hair?
    (1) Braid the hair in sections
    (2) Use a comb instead of a brush
    (3) Comb a small section at a time
    (4) Brush from the roots toward the ends

14. The nurse makes the assessment that the patient's feet are dirty. When planning to clean the patient's feet, the *most* effective intervention would be to:
    (1) Ask the resident to take a shower
    (2) Lubricate them with lotion to soften the dirt
    (3) Soak each foot in a basin with soap and water
    (4) Use an antiseptic to prevent a fungal infection

15. When making an occupied bed, it is *most* important for the nurse to:
    (1) Utilize new linen
    (2) Raise both side rails
    (3) Keep the patient covered
    (4) Place an incontinence pad on the draw sheet

16. When washing the perineal area of a male patient, what is the most important action by the nurse?
    (1) Handling the genitalia with a very light touch
    (2) Washing the scrotum before the shaft of the penis
    (3) Repositioning the foreskin after washing the penis
    (4) Cleansing down the length of the penis toward the glans

17. A patient is incontinent of urine and stool and is cognitively impaired. To BEST prevent skin breakdown in this patient, the nurse should:
    (1) Gently instruct the patient to call the nurse when soiled
    (2) Frequently check the perineal area and wash if necessary
    (3) Turn and position the patient every 2 hours
    (4) Place sheepskin on the bed and apply a diaper

18. Mr. Covert has a nasogastric tube inserted into the stomach. A daily intervention that would contribute to hygiene would include:
    (1) Replacing the positioning tape on the nose
    (2) Instilling 30 ml of water into the tube
    (3) Suctioning the oral pharynx
    (4) Lubricating the nares

19. When assessing pain, the nurse must recognize that the *most* subjective characteristic of pain is its:
    (1) Intensity
    (2) Duration
    (3) Location
    (4) Quality

20. Patients with chronic pain often have psychological adaptations. A psychological reaction to pain which the nurse should monitor for is:
    (1) Dyspnea
    (2) Depression
    (3) Hypertension
    (4) Self-splinting

21. The individual who generally requires the least amount of sleep is the:
    (1) Adolescent
    (2) Young adult
    (3) Older adult
    (4) Middle-age adult

22. To promote sleep, the nurse should encourage the patient to:
    (1) Exercise daily
    (2) Eat light meals
    (3) Drink a cup of tea
    (4) Review the day's events

23. A behavioral response to moderate pain that the nurse should assess for is:
    (1) Rapid, irregular breathing
    (2) Increased muscle tension
    (3) Self-splinting
    (4) Fatigue

24. During a clinic visit an elderly patient complains about cold feet. The nurse should:
    (1) Encourage the patient to wear warm socks
    (2) Instruct the patient in how to use a hot water bottle
    (3) Teach the patient to place a heating pad over the feet
    (4) Explain to the patient that this is normal in the elderly

25. A perioperative patient verbalizes that he is afraid of the pain he had with his last surgery. To help the patient deal with this fear, the nurse should:
    (1) Encourage the patient not to be afraid
    (2) Teach the patient relaxation techniques
    (3) Listen to the patient's concerns about pain
    (4) Inform him that he can have pain medication

26. In normal daily living, sleep is *most* often interfered with by:
    (1) Environmental noise
    (2) Emotional concerns
    (3) Room temperature
    (4) Body discomfort

27. Mr. Parker is in continuous pain from cancer that has metastasized to the bone. Pain medication provides little relief and he refuses to move. The nurse should plan to:
    (1) Reassure him that the nurses will not hurt him
    (2) Let him perform his own activities of daily living
    (3) Touch him gently when assisting with required care
    (4) Complete A.M. care quickly as possible when necessary

28. Pain perception is *most* influenced by the:
    (1) Duration of the stimulus
    (2) Characteristics of the pain
    (3) Activity of the cerebral cortex
    (4) Level of endorphins in the blood

29. The nurse understands that narcotic analgesics limit pain by:
    (1) Diminishing peripheral pain reception
    (2) Competing with receptors for sensory input

(3) Modifying the patient's perception of pain
(4) Closing the gating mechanism for impulse transmission

30. When planning care to relieve pain, the nurse could use an intervention that incorporates the gate control theory of pain such as:
    (1) Administering a narcotic
    (2) Talking with the patient
    (3) Applying a warm compress
    (4) Promoting rest and sleep

31. Cold is effective in reducing the discomfort associated with a local inflammatory response because it:
    (1) Anesthetizes nerve endings
    (2) Lowers tissue metabolism
    (3) Decreases venous return
    (4) Causes vasodilation

32. To best promote rest and sleep in the hospital for all patients, the nurse should:
    (1) Provide a backrub prior to sleep
    (2) Administer a sleeping medication
    (3) Turn the lights off at night
    (4) Encourage usual routines

33. A backrub promotes comfort and rest because it:
    (1) Causes vasodilation
    (2) Stimulates circulation
    (3) Increases O_2 to tissues
    (4) Relieves muscular tension

34. Heat effectively reduces discomfort at a local inflammatory site because it:
    (1) Limits capillary permeability
    (2) Decreases tissue metabolism
    (3) Promotes muscle relaxation
    (4) Provides local anesthesia

35. A patient is admitted with acute pain. When assessing the patient, which of the following signs should the nurse expect?
    (1) Decreased respiratory rate
    (2) Increased blood pressure
    (3) Constricted pupils
    (4) Flushed skin

Rationales

1. * (1) Diaphoresis is a profuse secretin of sweat which is associated with an elevated body temperature, physical exertion, or emotional stress. The secretions must be removed from the entire body to limit the growth of microorganisms and promote comfort; evaporation during the bed bath may help lower the patient's temperature.
   (2) This is inadequate; a complete bed bath is necessary.
   (3) This is unsafe; the patient needs immediate physical hygiene.
   (4) Same as #2.

2. (1) This would be used to store the dentures when the patient is sleeping.
   * (2) This provides privacy while the dentures are out of the mouth and supports the patient's dignity and self-esteem.

      (3) This supports the patient's physical needs.

      (4) The nurse must look at the patient to inspect the oral cavity.

3.   (1) This is too cool; this would promote chilling.

      (2) Same as #1.

 * (3) The temperature of bath water should be between 110 and 115°F to promote comfort, dilate blood vessels, and prevent chilling.

      (4) This is too hot; this would be uncomfortable and could injure tissue.

4.   (1) This provides for physical comfort.

 * (2) Perineal care is a private activity, and measures should be employed to provide privacy.

      (3) Same as #1.

      (4) Although this is a respectful, individualized approach, it does not address the patient's right to privacy during a procedure that exposes the genitalia.

5. * (1) These areas should be washed daily because they harbor the most microorganisms.

      (2) This would be a complete bed bath with assistance.

      (3) The axillary areas and the back must also be washed in a partial bed bath.

      (4) Same as #2.

6.   (1) This is contraindicated; *Non Per Os* (NPO) means nothing by mouth.

 * (2) When people are NPO, they tend to have dry mucous membranes and thick secretions on the tongue and gums; mouth care cleans the oral cavity.

      (3) Same as #1.

      (4) Although this may be done, the priority is direct physical care of the patient.

7.   (1) Friction from firm long strokes increases circulation.

      (2) A backrub and positioning in functional alignment promote rest and comfort.

      (3) Local massage and repositioning every 2 hours prevent decubitus ulcers.

 * (4) Rinsing flushes the skin with clean water which removes debris and soap residue.

8.   (1) Although some foods can cause halitosis, it is more often caused by poor oral hygiene, a local infection, or a systemic disease; brushing uses friction which most often effectively cleans the oral cavity.

 * (2) Halitosis is often caused by decaying food particles and gingivitis; brushing the teeth and tongue cleans the oral cavity and promotes healthy teeth and gums.

      (3) This is done after brushing the teeth and tongue; rinsing alone will not remove debris caught between the teeth.

      (4) Same as #3.

9.   (1) Conditioners moisturize the hair which makes the strands more supple, preventing tangles.

 * (2) Soap is drying because it removes natural secretions which keep the hair supple.

      (3) Braids organize the strands of hair which limits movement of hair into mats and tangles due to friction and pressure.

      (4) This distributes oils along hair shafts, keeping them supple and preventing tangles and matting.

10.   (1) This is an additional sheet which could add to the number of wrinkles; the purpose of a draw sheet is to keep the bottom sheet clean.
    * (2) Wrinkles exert pressure and friction against the skin, promoting the formation of decubitus ulcers.
      (3) A toe pleat prevents foot drop, not decubitus ulcers.
      (4) This is unnecessary unless the sheet is wet or dirty.

11.   (1) This is too cool and could cause chilling.
      (2) Same as #1.
      (3) Same as #1.
    * (4) Bath water should be between 110 and 115°F to promote comfort and prevent chilling.

12. * (1) The sun promotes loss of fluid from the skin, and the ultraviolet rays could cause a burn.
      (2) This is contraindicated; soap and water are irritating and drying because they remove natural secretions that lubricate the skin.
      (3) This exposes the skin to the sun which promotes drying.
      (4) Itchy areas should be patted, not rubbed, to prevent damage to tissues.

13.   (1) This should be done after the hair is combed and untangled.
      (2) Either a comb or a brush can be used.
    * (3) Separating the hair into small sections promotes ease in combing and limits discomfort.
      (4) When removing tangles, the hair should be grasped at the scalp and the loose ends combed; each stroke should start progressively higher than the preceding stroke up the shafts of hair strands.

14.   (1) This is not as effective as submerging the feet in soapy water.
      (2) This is done after the feet are clean to lubricate the skin.
    * (3) Soaking softens the skin and debris on the skin, between the toes, and under the toenails facilitating cleaning.
      (4) This requires a physician's order.

15.   (1) This is unnecessary unless the linens are wet or dirty.
      (2) This does not support correct body mechanics when working and puts excess stress on the nurse; the side rail may be lowered on the side the nurse is working.
    * (3) This supports privacy and dignity and prevents chilling.
      (4) This promotes the formation of decubitus ulcers; it should be used only during perineal care or for patients who are incontinent.

16.   (1) This would be stimulating and could precipitate a penile erection; a firm but gentle touch should be used.
      (2) This violates the principle of working from clean to dirty; the tip of the penis at the urethral meatus is washed first; bathing should then progress down the shaft of the penis, and then the scrotum is washed.
    * (3) This protects the head of the penis and prevents drying and irritation; if allowed to remain retracted, the tightening of the foreskin around the shaft of the penis could cause local edema and discomfort.
      (4) Cleaning should occur in the opposite direction, starting at the urinary meatus and then progressing down the shaft of the penis away from the urinary meatus.

17.   (1) This is unrealistic; a cognitively impaired patient would have difficulty following this instruction.

   * (2) When patients are incontinent, they should immediately be cleaned; feces contain digestive enzymes and urine contains ammonia and other irritating substances that cause skin breakdown.

    (3) Although important, the removal of warm moist, irritating excreta best prevents skin breakdown in the incontinent patient; turning may be necessary more frequently than every 2 hours in a patient at risk.

    (4) Sheepskin and an incontinence pad (the word "diaper" should be avoided) hold moisture next to the skin, and their use should be avoided.

18.   (1) It is unnecessary to do this daily; the tape should be reapplied if the nares become irritated or the tape becomes soiled.

    (2) After placement is established, this may be done to promote patency, not hygiene.

    (3) Suctioning is unnecessary; cleaning the oral cavity when necessary with a toothbrush, dental floss, mouthwash, and a lubricant is sufficient.

   * (4) This keeps the skin supple and prevents drying which limit the development of encrustations.

19. * (1) This is the most subjective characteristic of pain; a patient's perception of pain influences the descriptive report about the severity of pain.

    (2) This description is based on determining onset, periodicity, frequency, and duration; it is based on time frames which can be objectively measured by the patient.

    (3) This description is based on anatomical landmarks in the patient's attempt to localize the pain; it is less subjective than intensity.

    (4) Although subjective, it is less subjective than intensity. There is more consistency in the language used to describe types of pain; surgical pain is generally described as "sharp" and pain related to a heart attack is described as "crushing."

20.   (1) This is a physiological adaptation to a stress, not a psychological adaptation.

   * (2) Patients with chronic pain commonly experience depression; this is an adaptation to lack of control over relentless pain.

    (3) Same as #1.

    (4) This is a physical attempt to minimize pain.

21.   (1) Adolescents go through a growth spurt and need more sleep than the older adult.

    (2) Young adults may still be growing and need more sleep; they are usually very active and need more sleep than an older adult.

   * (3) Studies demonstrate that the older adult requires less sleep than people at any other developmental level.

    (4) These adults are usually involved with activities related to growing children; they also are investing time and effort in a career. This age requires more sleep than the older adult.

22. * (1) This contributes to physical and mental relaxation which reduces tension and promotes sleep.

    (2) The opposite is true. Moderate to heavy meals promote sleep; the body's energy is engaged in the process of digestion.

(3) Tea contains caffeine; caffeine contributes to wakefulness.

(4) This can cause an increase in tension; it can prevent a person from falling asleep.

23. (1) This is a physiological response to pain; pain generally activates the fight-or-flight mechanism of the general adaption syndrome (GAS). The GAS stimulates the sympathetic branch of the autonomic nervous system which results in these symptoms; this response provides for greater oxygen transport.

(2) GAS stimulates the sympathetic branch of the autonomic nervous system which results in these symptoms; it is a physiological response that prepares muscles for action.

* (3) This is a behavioral attempt to protect the area in pain and minimize stress and strain to the area, for example, supporting the area or leaning in the direction of the pain.

(4) This is a physical response to pain; emotional and physiological responses to pain can use a great deal of physical and emotional energy and leave a person fatigued.

24. * (1) This is the safest way to keep the feet warm; socks contain the heat around the feet that has been generated by the body.

(2) This is not as safe as socks; externally produced heat can burn the feet in elderly people who have reduced peripheral sensation.

(3) Same as #2.

(4) This ignores the patient's comfort needs.

25. (1) This denies the patient's fears.

(2) Although this may eventually be done, it does not allow the patient to discuss fears.

* (3) This supports the patient's need to verbalize the fears.

(4) This is false reassurance and cuts off communication; it does not recognize the patient's need to verbalize fears.

26. (1) While this can interfere with sleep, emotional concerns have proven most often to interfere with sleep.

* (2) This is suggested by studies; emotional concerns interfere with the patient's ability to relax the mind and body and fall asleep.

(3) Same as #1.

(4) Same as #1.

27. (1) This is false reassurance; this is something the nurse cannot promise.

(2) The patient refuses to move now and will probably avoid any self-care that requires movement.

* (3) This conveys that the nurse recognizes the patient's need to move slowly, gently, and carefully; avoiding quick and firm movements will contribute to the patient's comfort.

(4) This can intensify pain; also it can tire the patient which may intensify pain.

28. (1) Duration is one component of a description of pain once it is perceived.

(2) Characteristics of pain are the components of the description of pain once it is perceived.

* (3) This controls the higher levels of the perceptual aspects of pain.

(4) While endorphin levels influence pain perception, it is the activity of the cerebral cortex that controls the higher levels of the perceptual aspects of pain.

29. (1) Local anesthetics, not narcotics, produce loss of localized sensation by inhibiting nerve conduction and thus the perception of pain.
(2) This is the theory related to increasing distracting sensory input to inhibit painful stimuli perception.
* (3) Narcotics modify pain perception by acting on the higher centers of the brain to inhibit the perception of pain.
(4) Narcotics do not close synaptic gates; stimulation of large nerve fibers via methods such as transcutaneous electrical stimulation close synaptic gates.

30. (1) This acts on the higher centers of the brain to modify the perception of pain.
(2) This increases sensory input; distraction focuses attention on stimuli other than the pain.
* (3) This theory assumes that pain fibers originating in the peripheral areas of the body synapse in the gray matter of the dorsal horns of the spinal cord. Large nerve fibers stimulated by heat, cold, and touch transmit impulses through the same synapses as those that transmit pain; when larger fibers are stimulated, they close the gate to painful stimuli, and the perception of pain is reduced.
(4) Promoting rest and sleep includes efforts to reduce muscle tension. When muscle tension is reduced, pain also usually decreases; relaxation increases a sense of control that reduces anxiety, which in turn reduces pain perception.

31. * (1) Cold is a form of cutaneous stimulation that slows the nervous conduction of impulses which relaxes muscle tension, relieving pain.
(2) Although cold does lower tissue metabolism, this is not the physiologic response that reduces pain.
(3) Although this would occur with vasoconstriction, it is not the reason for pain relief.
(4) Application of cold causes vasoconstriction, not vasodilation.

32. (1) A backrub invades personal space and should be administered depending on a patient's need and preference; a backrub may be contraindicated in certain clinical situations such as a patient with a myocardial infarction.
(2) Sleeping medication should not be administered until all nondrug approaches fail to achieve sleep.
(3) In an unfamiliar environment turning the lights off can precipitate confusion or disorientation; a small light provides for visual cues if a person should awaken at night.
* (4) Usual routines meet self-identified needs and reduce anxiety because they provide a familiar pattern.

33. (1) The friction of a backrub causes heat which in turn causes vasodilation. Vasodilation improves circulation by bringing oxygen and nutrients to the area; these physiological effects do not promote comfort or rest.
(2) Same as #1.
(3) Same as #1.
* (4) Effleurage, applying long smooth strokes while moving the hands up and down the back without losing contact with the skin, has a relaxing and sedative effect. Its effect may be related to the gate control theory of pain relief; rubbing the back stimulates large muscle fiber groups which close the synaptic gates to pain or uncomfortable stimuli, permitting a perception of relaxation.

34. (1) Heat increases capillary vasodilation and permeability.
  (2) Heat increases, not decreases, tissue metabolism; heat causes vasodilation, facilitating the exchange of nutrients and waste products, which increases cellular metabolism.
  * (3) Heat is known to relax muscle spasms and the discomfort associated with muscle spasm; the mechanism is unknown.
  (4) Cold applications cause local anesthesia, not the application of heat.

35. (1) With acute pain the patient will have an increased respiratory rate.
  * (2) Sympathetic stimulation in response to the fight-or-flight mechanism increases vasomotor tone and peripheral vascular resistance, increasing the blood pressure.
  (3) In the general adaptation syndrome the pupils dilate to increase visual acuity.
  (4) Pallor is expected; peripheral vasoconstriction occurs in an effort to shift the blood supply from the periphery to the skeletal muscles, viscera, and brain.

MEETING PATIENT'S FLUID AND NUTRITIONAL NEEDS

This section encompasses questions related to basic fluid balance and nutrition. Specific questions focus on principles associated with therapeutic diets, enteral feedings, fluid and electrolyte balance, intake and output, feeding patients, vitamins, dehydration, essential minerals, total parenteral nutrition, intralipids, and medications associated with meeting nutritional needs.

Questions

1. A patient who drinks small amounts of fluid will:
   (1) Produce urine with a specific gravity of 1.020
   (2) Urinate small amounts at each voiding
   (3) Develop an atonic bladder
   (4) Have dark amber urine

2. A patient receiving chemotherapy is nauseated. When planning for this patient's nutritional needs, the nurse should:
   (1) Obtain an order for a full liquid diet
   (2) Withhold food by mouth until the nausea subsides
   (3) Provide meals and supplements as previously planned
   (4) Serve the ordered diet in small quantities frequently

3. When feeding Mr. Learner who has hemiparesis due to a stroke, the nurse should:
   (1) Ensure that food is either soft or pureed
   (2) Provide fluids with each bite to liquify the food
   (3) Allow him time to empty his mouth between spoonfuls
   (4) Promote conversation since meals should be a social time

4. What should the nurse do FIRST when caring for a patient on intake and output?
   (1) Remove the pitcher of water from the bedside
   (2) Post an intake and output sign over the patient's bed
   (3) Explain the meaning of intake and output to the patient
   (4) Measure the amount of fluid the patient drinks and voids

5. When urine output is less than fluid intake, the nurse can expect the patient to:
   (1) Gain weight
   (2) Void frequently

(3) Become jaundiced
(4) Experience nausea

6. To prevent burns during mealtime in clients with mental and physical impairments, the nurse should:
(1) Assist patients with warm drinks
(2) Use plastic instead of metal utensils
(3) Serve unsteady patients just cold drinks
(4) Wait until the food is cool before serving

7. When a patient drinks 9 ounces of milk, which of the following calculations should the nurse enter on the intake and output record?
(1) 30 ml
(2) 90 ml
(3) 240 ml
(4) 270 ml

8. An obese patient is on a 1000-calorie diet. The action which is LEAST therapeutic is:
(1) Recognizing when the patient has lost weight
(2) Encouraging the patient to chew and eat slowly
(3) Identifying low-calorie snacks that the patient can eat
(4) Teaching the patient to avoid starches on the meal tray

9. What is the most accurate way to measure the amount of urine in a drainage collection bag?
(1) With a urometer
(2) With a marked graduate
(3) By the markings on the bag
(4) By emptying it in a bed pan

10. When the amount of calories ingested is not sufficient for the patient's basal metabolic rate, the patient will:
(1) Become dehydrated
(2) Develop anorexia
(3) Lose weight
(4) Sleep more

11. To avoid trauma to the oral mucous membranes by hot food being served to a cognitively impaired patient, the nurse should:
(1) Request a menu that includes many cold foods
(2) Mix the hot food with appropriate cold food
(3) Touch the food to test its temperature
(4) Wait for the hot food to cool down

12. A patient becomes easily confused. To meet his nutritional needs, the most appropriate nursing intervention would be:
(1) Assisting him to eat
(2) Feeding him his meals
(3) Explaining where everything is on the tray
(4) Encouraging his family to take turns feeding him

13. To maintain *normal* fluid balance, how much fluid should the nurse give a patient during 24 hours?
(1) 500 ml
(2) 1000 ml
(3) 2000 ml
(4) 3000 ml

14. A patient who had a heart attack because of atherosclerotic plaques should obtain protein by ingesting:
    (1) White meats
    (2) Legumes
    (3) Shrimp
    (4) Milk

15. A patient's pulse is full and bounding. The nurse should:
    (1) Measure the urine specific gravity
    (2) Lower the head of the bed
    (3) Monitor the serum glucose
    (4) Check the rate of the IV

16. A patient with a deficiency in vitamin K should be assessed for:
    (1) Muscle cramps
    (2) Signs of infection
    (3) Bleeding tendencies
    (4) Cardiac dysrhythmias

17. When caring for a patient with a draining decubitus ulcer, the nurse recognizes which of the following losses as being most significant?
    (1) Fluid
    (2) Weight
    (3) Protein
    (4) Leukocytes

18. As a result of being on a low-calorie diet, all patients will:
    (1) Break down adipose tissue for energy
    (2) Have a decreased body metabolism
    (3) Have decreased energy levels
    (4) Require vitamin supplements

19. An age group that has the highest energy requirements is:
    (1) Birth to 1 year old
    (2) 3 to 5 years old
    (3) 13 to 19 years old
    (4) Over 65 years old

20. A patient is admitted with a diagnosis of dehydration. When assessing the patient, which of the following symptoms would support this diagnosis?
    (1) Poor skin turgor
    (2) Straw colored urine
    (3) Decreased heart rate
    (4) Urine specific gravity of 1.015

21. Iron absorption is facilitated by vitamin:
    (1) D
    (2) C
    (3) A
    (4) K

22. A patient is on a low-sodium diet. The nurse should encourage the patient to ingest:
    (1) Milk
    (2) Fruit
    (3) Bread
    (4) Vegetables

23. Which of the following breakfast foods would contribute the most to the healing of a patient's decubitus ulcer?
    (1) Oatmeal
    (2) Bran flakes

(3) Poached eggs
(4) French toast

24. An essential vitamin for a patient with anemia would be:
    (1) Ascorbic acid
    (2) Riboflavin
    (3) Folic acid
    (4) Thiamin

25. When a patient is receiving total parenteral nutrition (TPN) and intralipids, the nurse MUST administer the intralipids:
    (1) Via an infusion pump
    (2) Through a separate line
    (3) After the total parenteral nutrition is completed
    (4) Piggybacked into the proximal port of the TPN catheter

26. The patient is on a full liquid diet. Which of the following foods should be removed from the diet?
    (1) Ice cream
    (2) Prune juice
    (3) Cream of wheat
    (4) Raspberry [Jello]

27. Increasing the flow rate of total parenteral nutrition above the prescribed rate is dangerous because it can result in:
    (1) Infection
    (2) Hypoglycemia
    (3) Osmotic diuresis
    (4) Dumping syndrome

28. Once an intermittent gastrostomy tube feeding is completed, the nurse should:
    (1) Insert 30 ml of air into the tube
    (2) Gently instill 30 ml of water
    (3) Check the dressing site
    (4) Encourage activity

29. Supplemental iron is most needed by:
    (1) Elderly men
    (2) Growing children
    (3) Menstruating women
    (4) Active adolescents

30. A factor related to normal aging that influences the nutritional status of elderly people is a:
    (1) Decreased need for a balanced diet
    (2) Greater production of gastric acid
    (3) Deterioration in taste perception
    (4) Magnified need for kilocalories

31. To maintain life, the most important nutrients are:
    (1) Carbohydrates
    (2) Vitamins
    (3) Proteins
    (4) Fluids

32. The individual with the GREATEST need for calcium is a:
    (1) Postmenopausal woman
    (2) School-age child
    (3) Pregnant woman
    (4) Working man

Rationales

1. (1) Reduced fluid intake will produce a concentrated urine with a specific gravity higher than 1.025.
    (2) This is not true; the bladder will still fill to the patient's normal capacity before there is a perceived need to void.
    (3) This is caused by a neurological problem; it is a loss of the sensation of fullness which leads to distension from overfilling.
    * (4) This is the color of urine that the nurse can expect when fluid intake is below 1500 to 2000 ml per day; the urine is concentrated.

2. (1) This is unnecessary; it will not reduce the nausea.
    (2) The patient could be nauseated for a long period of time; adequate food and fluid must be ingested to meet physiological needs.
    (3) Meals served with regular-size portions can be overwhelming for the patient experiencing nausea.
    * (4) This establishes small realistic goals for the patient without being overwhelming.

3. (1) This may not be necessary; the patient may only need more time to thoroughly chew food.
    (2) This would increase the risk of aspiration; fluid is more difficult to control than food when swallowing.
    * (3) This minimizes food buildup in the mouth; also it does not rush the patient.
    (4) This is unsafe; the patient can easily aspirate when talking with food in the mouth.

4. (1) This could upset the patient if the procedure were not explained first.
    (2) This violates a patient's right to privacy; signs directing the staff should not be posted at the bedside where they can be seen and violate patient confidentiality.
    * (3) Before any procedure is implemented, the patient has the right to know what is being done and why; knowledge increases compliance.
    (4) This would be done after intake and output is explained to the patient.

5. * (1) Fluid has mass; when fluid is retained, the patient will gain weight. A patient can gain from 6 to 8 pounds before edema can be identified through inspection.
    (2) The opposite is true.
    (3) This is related to impaired liver and biliary function, not extracellular fluid excess.
    (4) This is not a common sign of extracellular fluid excess.

6. * (1) Patients with mental and physical deficits need assistance with warm drinks; this prevents burns from scalding.
    (2) This will not prevent spilling hot liquids; plastic utensils need to be used only in isolation.
    (3) Patients have a right to have a variety of foods presented at different temperatures; this would violate a patient's rights.
    (4) Hot foods should be served hot, and cold foods should be served cold.

7. (1) This is only 1 ounce.
    (2) This is only 3 ounces.
    (3) This is only 8 ounces.
    * (4) This is equal to 9 ounces.

8. (1) This is supportive; progress should be recognized to provide for motivation.
    (2) This is supportive; it makes a meal take longer and allows more time for the body to feel full.
    (3) This is supportive; it helps reduce caloric intake.
  * (4) This is inappropriate. The patient is receiving a special diet that has been carefully calculated; all food on the tray should be eaten.

9. (1) This is used to measure the specific gravity of urine, not the volume of urine.
  * (2) This is a special container with volume markings on the side for measuring fluid; of all the options it is the most accurate.
    (3) This is not as accurate as using a marked graduate because the plastic stretches and makes the marking inaccurate.
    (4) Bedpans are designed to collect excreta when a person cannot use a toilet or commode, not measure urine volume.

10. (1) This occurs when fluid intake is insufficient, not when calories are insufficient.
    (2) This is a loss of appetite which usually contributes to insufficient intake, not the result of insufficient intake.
  * (3) When calories are insufficient to meet metabolic needs, the body catabolizes fat, and as a result the patient will lose weight.
    (4) This is not directly related; however, a patient may easily tire if anemic from an inappropriate diet.

11. (1) Patients have a right to make their own menu selections within the ordered diet.
    (2) Foods should not be mixed; they should be served separately so they retain their own flavor and texture.
    (3) This would contaminate the food; a food thermometer designed for this purpose should be used, not a finger.
  * (4) This is the most safe and practical action; once hot food loses some of its heat, it will be safe to eat.

12. * (1) Providing assistance will keep the patient focused on the task of eating.
    (2) This is unnecessary; this would contribute to feelings of dependence.
    (3) This will not keep the patient focused on eating during the meal; although it is something the nurse may initially do to orient the patient, the patient may forget or not understand the explanation.
    (4) While helpful, it is the responsibility of the staff to care for the patient, not the family members.

13. (1) This is inadequate intake to maintain life.
    (2) Same as #1.
  * (3) This is an average daily intake necessary to maintain normal fluid balance.
    (4) This is more than the body needs for normal fluid balance.

14. (1) White meat contains less fat than red meat; however, white meat contains more fat than legumes.
  * (2) Legumes, such as beans, peas, and lentils, contain the least amount of cholesterol and fat of the options presented and are high in protein which is necessary for tissue regeneration.
    (3) Although shrimp is a protein source, it is high in cholesterol which should be avoided because it contributes to plaque formation.
    (4) Milk contains fat which contributes to plaque formation in atherosclerosis.

15.   (1) This reflects the concentrating ability of the kidneys, not the cardiovascular system.

      (2) A full bounding pulse may indicate hypervolemia; in a compromised patient, lowering the head of the bed could impede respirations and would therefore be contraindicated.

      (3) A full, bounding pulse is not related to hyper- or hypoglycemia; a weak thready pulse, not a full bounding pulse, will indicate hypotension and shock and are late signs of diabetic ketoacidosis. Bradycardia, not a full bounding pulse, is a symptom of hypoglycemia.

  * (4) IV solutions are administered directly into the intravascular compartment; if the IV flow rate is excessive, it could cause a full bounding pulse.

16.   (1) Calcium contributes to neuromuscular excitability, and therefore lowered calcium levels can result in muscle cramps and tetany.

      (2) Vitamins A and C help build resistance to infection.

  * (3) Vitamin K is essential for prothrombin formation and blood clotting; if a patient is deficient in vitamin K, the patient will experience a prolonged clotting time and be prone to bleeding.

      (4) A deficiency of vitamin B_1 (thiamin), not vitamin K, can result in tachycardia and cardiac enlargement; deficiencies in calcium, magnesium, and potassium can also contribute to cardiac problems.

17.   (1) While fluid is lost from a draining decubitus ulcer, it is the loss of protein in that fluid that has the most serious implication.

      (2) Weight loss is related to inadequate caloric intake, not the presence of a decubitus ulcer.

  * (3) Protein loss is a serious concern when a patient has a draining decubitus ulcer. A patient can loose as much as 50 grams of protein daily from a draining decubitus ulcer; this is a large percentage of the normal daily requirement of 60 grams of protein for women and 70 grams of protein for men. Patients with draining decubitus ulcers should ingest two to four times the normal daily requirements of protein to rebuild epidermal tissue.

      (4) Leukocyte counts increase in response to the threat of infection; if the decubitus ulcer is infected, the leukocyte count will increase, not decrease. Decreased white blood cell levels are a response to bone marrow depression caused by a stress other than a decubitus ulcer.

18. * (1) When the number of calories ingested does not meet the body's energy requirements, the patient will catabolize body fat for energy and lose weight.

      (2) Metabolism relates to the biochemical reactions that take place within the body to meet energy needs; metabolism will increase and decrease in response to the energy demands placed on the body, not as a result of a low-calorie diet.

      (3) Not all people experience a decrease in energy levels in response to a low-calorie diet, whereas all individuals will break down adipose tissue for energy if caloric intake is insufficient to meet metabolic needs. Age, body size, body and environmental temperatures, growth, sex, nutritional state, emotional state, and even food intake will affect energy levels.

      (4) A well-balanced low-calorie diet should contain adequate vitamins requiring no supplementation.

19. * (1) During the first year of life the infant grows at the faster pace than at any other developmental stage; infants double their birth weight by 6 months and triple their birth weight during the first year.

    (2) The preschool child's (3- to 5-year-old) growth rate is slower than it was during the first year of life; the preschool child gains only another 7 to 12 pounds in addition to the four times the birth weight gained during the first three years.

    (3) While the adolescent goes through a dramatic physical growth spurt that reflects significant changes in height, weight, dentition, and skeletal and sexual development, it is not as spectacular as the growth rate seen in the first year of life, during which the infant triples the birth weight.

    (4) No physical growth occurs when a person is over 65 years of age; different parts of the body begin to degenerate, and functions slow.

20. * (1) "Tissue turgor" refers to normal skin fullness or the ability of the skin and underlying tissue to return to their regular position after being pinched and lifted. When there is poor skin turgor due to dehydration, the skin remains pinched or "tented" for a longer period of time than well-hydrated skin after it is released.

    (2) This is the expected color of urine, and it indicates that the patient is probably in fluid balance.

    (3) The heart rate would increase and the pulse would be weak and thready because of hypovolemia.

    (4) This is within the normal range of 1.010 to 1.025; if the patient is dehydrated, the specific gravity would be over 1.025.

21.   (1) Vitamin D is essential for adequate absorption and utilization of calcium in bone and tooth growth; it does not facilitate the absorption of iron.

  * (2) Ascorbic acid (vitamin C) helps to change dietary iron to a form which can be absorbed by the body.

    (3) Vitamin A is essential for growth and maintenance of epithelial tissue, maintenance of night vision, and promotion of resistance to infection, not the absorption of iron.

    (4) Vitamin K is essential for the formation of prothrombin which prevents bleeding, not the absorption of iron.

22.   (1) Whole milk depending upon the brand has approximately 6 to 130 milligrams of sodium per 8 ounces.

  * (2) As a food group, fresh fruits contain the least amount of sodium per serving than the other options presented; most fresh fruits such as apples, pears, bananas, peaches, and cantaloupe contain under 10 milligrams of sodium per serving.

    (3) White bread depending upon the brand has approximately 55 to 225 milligrams of sodium per slice.

    (4) Fresh vegetables such as peas, beans, carrots, broccoli, cauliflower, corn, and celery contain approximately 40 milligrams of sodium per serving.

23.   (1) This nutrient does not contain protein which is essential for building cells and therefore wound healing.

    (2) Same as #1.

  * (3) Each egg contains 6 to 8 grams protein; protein contains amino acids necessary for building cells and therefore wound healing.

    (4) Although in French toast the bread is coated with an egg mixture, it does not contain as much protein as two eggs.

24.   (1) Vitamin C mainly functions to promote collagen formation, enhance iron absorption, and maintain capillary wall integrity.

      (2) Vitamin B_2 functions as a coenzyme in the metabolism of carbohydrates, fats, amino acids, and alcohol.

   * (3) Vitamin B_9 promotes the maturation of red blood cells.

      (4) Vitamin B_1 performs as a coenzyme in the metabolism of carbohydrates, fats, amino acids, and alcohol.

25.   (1) Because an intralipid solution is a concentrated source of nonprotein kilocalories, it would be desirable for an infusion pump to be used; however, an infusion pump does not have to be used because the solution can flow by gravity.

   * (2) If mixed with a dextrose–amino acid solution, the fat emulsion will break down; the solutions must not be administered through the same line.

      (3) The solutions can be run at the same time but through different lines.

      (4) This would cause the fat emulsion to break down.

26.   (1) This food changes its state from a solid to a liquid at room temperature.

      (2) This is a fluid and is permitted on a full liquid diet.

   * (3) This is considered solid food and is not permitted on a full liquid diet.

      (4) Same as #1.

27.   (1) Infection is unrelated to flow rate; infection is related to inadequate surgical asepsis.

      (2) Because of the high glucose load of total parenteral nutrition (TPN), hyperglycemia, not hypoglycemia, could result.

   * (3) The hypertonic TPN solution pulls intracellular and interstitial fluid into the intravascular compartment; the increased blood volume increases circulation to the kidneys, raising urinary output.

      (4) This could occur with a tube feeding, not TPN.

28.   (1) This is contraindicated; instilling fluid, not air, following a feeding limits air in the stomach which can cause distention.

   * (2) This flushes the tube preventing future blockage from a buildup of formula along the sides of the lumen of the tube.

      (3) This is not necessarily part of the procedure for administering a gastrostomy tube feeding. Checking the dressing site should be done routinely such as every 4 hours or every shift; placement of the tube should be assessed prior to the feeding.

      (4) After a gastrostomy tube feeding, the patient should remain in a sitting or slightly elevated right lateral position for 30 minutes to limit the risk of aspiration.

29.   (1) Supplemental iron is unnecessary for this group of people.

      (2) Supplemental iron is unnecessary in growing children (1 to 13 years); infants (birth to 1 year) who are breastfed need some iron supplementation from 4 to 12 months of age, and formula-fed infants need iron supplementation throughout the first year of life.

   * (3) Iron is essential to the formation of hemoglobin, a component of red blood cells, which is lost in menstrual blood.

      (4) Same as #1.

30.   (1) The need for foods from all food groups continues throughout life.

      (2) Gastric secretions decrease, not increase, with aging.

* (3) Taste perception decreases because of atrophy of the taste buds and a reduced sense of smell; sweet and salty tastes are lost first.

(4) The need for kilocalories (calories) decreases because of the lower metabolic rate and the decrease in physical activity associated with the elderly.

31.   (1) Although important, the body can survive longer without this nutrient than it can without water.

(2) Same as #1.

(3) Same as #1.

* (4) The most basic nutrient need is water; 57 percent of the body of an average healthy male is water. Women have a smaller percentage than men because they have proportionately more fat. All body processes require an adequate fluid balance in the body.

32.   (1) Although postmenopausal women can benefit from calcium supplementation to prevent osteoporosis, the need is not as high as in the pregnant woman.

(2) This group of individuals does not have an increased need for calcium; an adequate intake of milk and dairy products will meet minimum daily requirements for calcium.

* (3) Calcium should be increased 50 percent to an intake of 1.2 grams per day to provide calcium for fetal tooth and bone development; this is essential during the third trimester when fetal bones are mineralized.

(4) Same as #2.

THE USE OF BODY MECHANICS AND MEETING PATIENTS' ALIGNMENT AND MOBILITY NEEDS

This section encompasses questions related to the prevention of complications and the maintenance and restoration of musculoskeletal function. Questions focus on knowledge, principles, and devices related to the prevention of decubitus ulcers, contractures, and other hazards of immobility. Additional questions test principles associated with body alignment, transfer, range of motion, ambulation, positioning, and dressing and undressing.

Questions

1. During the transfer of a patient from the bed to a chair, what should the nurse say to the patient to determine adaptation to standing?
   (1) "Do you feel light-headed or dizzy?"
   (2) "Would you prefer to return to bed?"
   (3) "When was the last time you were out of bed?"
   (4) "How long would you like to sit in the chair?"

2. Sheepskin contributes to decubitus ulcer prevention primarily by:
   (1) Absorbing urine
   (2) Minimizing friction
   (3) Eliminating pressure
   (4) Keeping the skin warm

3. To best prevent a decubitus ulcer in an elderly person, the nurse should provide:
   (1) An air mattress
   (2) A daily bed bath

   (3) A high-protein diet
   (4) An indwelling urinary catheter

4. The LEAST helpful intervention by the nurse to safely move a patient from a bed to a chair is:
   (1) Allowing the patient to sit on the bed prior to transfer
   (2) Positioning the chair so the seat faces the bedside
   (3) Seeking another person to help with the transfer
   (4) Ensuring that the wheels of the bed are locked

5. An unconscious patient should be positioned with the:
   (1) Hips in external rotation
   (2) Fingers slightly flexed
   (3) Head hyperextended
   (4) Legs in adduction

6. When providing range-of-motion exercises, touching the thumb to the small fifth finger of the same hand is called:
   (1) Flexion
   (2) Adduction
   (3) Extension
   (4) Opposition

7. Mr. Gunter is visually impaired and is afraid to walk because he may trip and fall. The nurse's *best* intervention would be to:
   (1) Describe his environment to him
   (2) Instruct him to wear his glasses
   (3) Encourage him to walk around his bed
   (4) Assist him with ambulating while hospitalized

8. To safely transfer an obese patient who has paraplegia to a chair, the nurse should:
   (1) Pivot the patient
   (2) Utilize a pull sheet
   (3) Use a mechanical lift
   (4) Get another nurse to assist

9. The most therapeutic exercise that can be done by a patient on bed rest is:
   (1) Active range of motion
   (2) Passive range of motion
   (3) Active-assistive exercises
   (4) Contracting and relaxing muscles

10. A serious complication that can develop as a result of prolonged wheelchair use is:
   (1) Respiratory infections
   (2) Urinary tract infections
   (3) Thrombophlebitis of the legs
   (4) Extension contractures of the hips

11. A patient with one-sided weakness (hemiparesis) needs help transferring to a chair. To do this safely, the nurse should:
   (1) Stand on the patient's weak side
   (2) Keep the patient's feet together
   (3) Pivot the patient on the strong leg
   (4) Hold the patient under both forearms

12. To prevent injury when applying a restraint, the nurse should *first:*
   (1) Secure the strap in a double knot
   (2) Tie the restraint to the bed frame
   (3) Position the patient in functional alignment
   (4) Pad the patient's bony prominences with sheepskin

13. To promote safety when dressing and undressing a patient, the nurse should:
    (1) Remove clothing from the weaker side first
    (2) Support joints when moving an extremity
    (3) Put clothing on the stronger side first
    (4) Leave the bed rails up during dressing

14. A contracture is most often caused by:
    (1) Excessive pressure
    (2) Joint disease
    (3) Inactivity
    (4) Aging

15. The primary purpose of an eggcrate mattress is to:
    (1) Absorb moisture
    (2) Provide a soft surface
    (3) Support the body in alignment
    (4) Distribute pressure over a larger area

16. The nurse is transferring a patient from the bed to a chair using a mechanical lift. As the nurse raises the lift off the bed, the patient begins to panic and scream. The nurse should:
    (1) Lower the patient back onto the bed
    (2) Quickly continue and say, "It's almost over."
    (3) Say, "Relax" and slowly continue with the transfer
    (4) Stop the lift from rising until the patient regains control

17. The position that would contribute to the development of a decubitus ulcer in the sacral area is the:
    (1) Sim's position
    (2) Prone position
    (3) Lateral position
    (4) High-Fowler's position

18. The nurse assists a patient with range-of-motion exercises. The action of closing the hand into a fist is called:
    (1) Flexion
    (2) Adduction
    (3) Supination
    (4) Opposition

19. When assisting a blind patient to walk, the nurse should:
    (1) Stand behind the patient and provide directions
    (2) Instruct the patient to hold onto the nurse's arm
    (3) Walk on the side while holding the patient's elbow
    (4) Walk in front while the patient uses the corridor handrail

20. Range-of-motion exercises:
    (1) Prevent the formation of decubitus ulcers
    (2) Minimize the effects of immobility
    (3) Provide for aerobic conditioning
    (4) Contribute to muscle growth

21. To safely move a patient with slight hemiparesis from the bed to a wheelchair, the nurse should:
    (1) Lower just one side rail on the patient's bed
    (2) Lock the wheels of the bed and the wheelchair
    (3) Get another person to assist with the transfer
    (4) Close the door and pull the curtain around the bed

22. While lying in the dorsal recumbent position, a patient's leg externally rotates. What equipment should the nurse use to prevent external rotation?
    (1) Foot board
    (2) Bed cradle
    (3) Trochanter roll
    (4) Elastic stockings

23. A patient with the highest risk of developing a decubitus ulcer is the patient who:
    (1) Uses a reclining wheelchair
    (2) Is on bed rest but is able to move
    (3) Utilizes crutches to ambulate
    (4) Is ambulatory but is confused

24. The nurse assists a patient with range-of-motion exercises. The action of rolling the leg and foot toward the midline is:
    (1) Internal rotation
    (2) Lateral flexion
    (3) Adduction
    (4) Inversion

25. Mrs. Tack is afraid of falling and gets anxious when it is time to get out of bed (OOB) to a chair. The *best* action by the nurse to reduce the patient's anxiety would be to:
    (1) Use a mechanical lift
    (2) Transfer her at her own pace
    (3) Explain that she will not fall
    (4) Allow her to decide when to get OOB

26. Flotation pads or gel cushions are used to:
    (1) Deliver heat
    (2) Distribute body weight
    (3) Permit air to circulate
    (4) Prevent trapping moisture

27. To prevent a patient from developing contractures, the nurse should:
    (1) Support the joints with pillows
    (2) Transfer the patient to a chair twice a day
    (3) Turn and reposition the patient every 2 hours
    (4) Teach the patient to perform active range of motion

28. Mrs. Blue had a stroke 3 days ago and has a left hemiparesis. When dressing Mrs. Blue, the nurse should plan to:
    (1) Put Mrs. Blue's left sleeve on first
    (2) Encourage Mrs. Blue to dress by herself
    (3) Instruct Mrs. Blue to wear clothes with zippers
    (4) Tell Mrs. Blue to get clothes with buttons in the front

29. When transferring a patient from the bed to a chair, the nurse sits the patient on the side of the bed for several minutes primarily to:
    (1) Allow the patient to regain energy expended while siting
    (2) Enable the body to adapt to a drop in blood pressure
    (3) Provide time for the heart rate to return to normal
    (4) Permit the patient to take several deep breaths

30. When positioning a patient, the *most* important principle of body mechanics is:
    (1) Elevating the arms on pillows
    (2) Making the patient comfortable
    (3) Maintaining functional alignment
    (4) Keeping the head higher than the heart

31. Which of the following would be *most* effective in limiting moisture under the patient:
    (1) Bath blanket
    (2) Incontinence pad
    (3) Sheepskin pad
    (4) Alternating air mattress

32. The main cause of decubitus ulcers is:
    (1) Gravity
    (2) Pressure
    (3) Skin breakdown
    (4) Cellular necrosis

33. The nurse is assisting a patient with range-of-motion exercises. The action of turning the palm of the hand up toward the ceiling is:
    (1) Extension
    (2) Inversion
    (3) Supination
    (4) Circumduction

34. When positioning a patient in a lateral position, which of the following actions by the nurse would MOST contribute to the patient's functional alignment?
    (1) Using a foot board
    (2) Utilizing a bed cradle
    (3) Putting a pillow under the upper leg
    (4) Positioning a pillow under the waist

35. The nurse provides passive range of motion primarily to prevent which of the following complications?
    (1) Joint contractures
    (2) Decubitus ulcers
    (3) Muscle atrophy
    (4) Muscle spasms

36. The most effective independent nursing measure to prevent contractures in an immobilized patient would be to:
    (1) Apply a hand and wrist splint
    (2) Place an eggcrate mattress on the bed
    (3) Turn from side to side every 2 hours
    (4) Position the patient in functional alignment

Rationales

1. * (1) This assesses the patient's response to standing; it seeks subjective information directly from the patient who is the primary source.
    (2) This does not assess the patient's response to standing.
    (3) Same as #2.
    (4) Same as #2.

2. (1) It is not designed to absorb urine; wet lamb's wool will contribute to skin breakdown.
    * (2) Soft tufts of lamb's wool reduce friction and allow air to circulate under the patient.
    (3) Turning the patient off a body part is the most effective measure to relieve pressure; relieving pressure is not the rationale for using lamb's wool.
    (4) It helps to keep skin cool by allowing air to circulate through the tufts of lamb's wool.

3. * (1) This is effective because it distributes body weight over a large surface and reduces pressure over body prominences.
   (2) While bathing removes secretions and promotes clean dry skin, it can also be very drying which can compromise skin integrity.
   (3) Protein is the body's only source of nitrogen and is essential for building, repairing, or replacing body tissue; it does not prevent decubitus ulcers.
   (4) This should never be used to prevent a decubitus ulcer; however, a catheter may be used to prevent contamination of a decubitus ulcer once it is present.

4. (1) This contributes to safety; it allows time for the patient's body to adjust to orthostatic hypotension, preventing dizziness and falls.
   * (2) This is unsafe; the arm of the chair should be next to the side of the bed. This enables the nurse to easily move the patient using the pivot transfer.
   (3) This contributes to safety; two people provide a wider base of support when transferring a patient.
   (4) This contributes to safety; it prevents the bed from slipping out from under the patient as the patient pushes off the bed when rising to a standing position.

5. (1) This is not a position of normal alignment and, if allowed over a period of time, can result in a contracture that causes an unbalanced gait.
   * (2) This is a position of normal alignment; fingers should be maintained in this position with the use of splints or hand rolls to prevent flexion contractures of the fingers.
   (3) This is not a position of normal alignment; this abnormal position is usually a response to conditions affecting the central nervous system that cause spasms of the neck muscles and painful hyperextension of the head.
   (4) This is not a position of normal alignment. This is when the legs are moved toward the medial position; adduction contractures result in limited loco-motion and a scissor gait.

6. (1) Closing the fingers into a fist is flexion.
   (2) Bringing the fingers in alignment next to one another is adduction.
   (3) Straightening the finger joints is extension.
   * (4) This is the correct term to explain this action.

7. (1) This will help, but it will not prevent an accident; it does not address the patient's fear.
   (2) While glasses may help improve vision, this action does not address the patient's fear.
   (3) This is limiting; the problem is not mobility but fear of falling.
   * (4) This will reduce the patient's fear because the nurse is providing for the patient's physical safety.

8. (1) This is unsafe; a patient with paraplegia is unable to support weight on the legs to transfer.
   (2) This is unsafe; this is used by two or more people to move a patient up in bed, not to transfer a patient.
   * (3) This is the safest method to transfer an obese patient with paraplegia; the safety harness used during transfer provides support.
   (4) This is unsafe; an obese, dependent patient is too heavy and unstable for even two or three people to transfer to a chair without a mechanical lift.

9. * (1) This is preferable because it is an isotonic exercise that causes muscle contraction; this increases joint mobility, circulation, and muscle tone because the patient actively moves the joints through full range of motion.
    (2) This is when a joint is moved by a source other than the muscles articulating to the joint; it puts a joint through full range and prevents contractures, but does not increase muscle tone because the muscles are not contracting and relaxing.
    (3) This is when the patient attempts active range of motion and receives some support and assistance from the nurse; this does not provide for as much isotonic exercise as active range of motion.
    (4) This is isometric not isotonic exercise; it is contracting and relaxing a muscle without moving the joint; this improves muscle tone but does not put joints through range of motion.

10. (1) As long as a patient can cough and deep breathe, respiratory complications can be minimized even if a patient is confined to a wheelchair.
    (2) This is more of a problem when a patient is immobilized on bed rest rather than in a wheelchair; when on bed rest, not when in a wheelchair, the patient experiences urinary reflux which in turn causes distension of the renal pelvis resulting in pyelonephritis.
    * (3) This is true because decreased muscular contraction and hip flexion can result in venous stasis and hypercoagulability.
    (4) Flexion contractures, not extension contractures, are a concern with prolonged wheelchair use.

11. (1) This is unsafe; when transferring a patient, the nurse stands in front of the patient.
    (2) This is unsafe; keeping the feet apart provides a wide base of support which improves stability.
    * (3) This is a safe method to transfer a patient; it avoids extra unnecessary movement by directly transferring a patient to the chair while supporting body weight on the stronger leg.
    (4) When not using a transfer belt, place both hands under the patient's axillary areas and around the shoulder blades. Just using the arms places strain on the shoulder joints and is unsafe.

12. (1) This is unsafe; restraints are always tied in slip knots for easy release in an emergency.
    (2) This is important; however, functional alignment comes first.
    * (3) This is the first action; functional alignment positions muscles, joints, and bones in natural alignment, minimizing stress and strain on these structures.
    (4) Same as #2.

13. (1) This is an incorrect action; the stronger side has greater range of motion and should be dressed last and undressed first.
    * (2) Joints should always be supported when moving to reduce unnecessary strain; moving an unsupported joint can cause an injury to that joint.
    (3) Same as #1.
    (4) This is unnecessary if the nurse is at the bedside to provide for safety.

14. (1) This causes decubitus ulcers; immobility causes contractures.
    (2) Joint diseases can contribute to contractures; however, immobiity is generally the cause of contractures, not a disease process.

* (3) When a person is inactive, flexion muscles contract and extension muscles relax, causing flexion muscles to shorten and extender muscles to lengthen resulting in a contracture.

   (4) Aging does not cause a contracture; inactivity causes contractures.

15.   (1) The purpose is to distribute weight, not absorb moisture. In the event that it gets wet, it should be discarded; moisture against the skin can contribute to skin breakdown.

   (2) The purpose is to distribute weight, not provide a soft surface.

   (3) Pillows and wedges are used to keep the body in functional alignment, not an eggcrate mattress.

* (4) Intermittent raised areas on the mattress help to evenly distribute body weight over the entire surface.

16. * (1) This action recognizes the cause of the anxiety and responds to the source.

   (2) This denies the patient's fears and can intensify the anxiety.

   (3) Same as #2.

   (4) This leaves the patient up in the air, which can intensify the anxiety.

17.   (1) The Sim's position avoids pressure on the sacral area; weight is on the anterior ilium, the humerus, and clavicle.

   (2) The prone position avoids pressure on the sacral area; prone is lying on the abdomen.

   (3) In the lateral position pressure is off the sacral area; the body is side-lying with weight on the dependent hip and shoulder.

* (4) In this position most of the weight is placed on the sacral area; this causes sacral pressure.

18. * (1) This is the correct term for this action.

   (2) This is not the correct term for this action; adduction is when a body part is moved medially or together and beyond if possible.

   (3) This is not the correct term for this action; supination is when the lower arm and hand is turned so that the palm is up.

   (4) This is not the correct term for this action; opposition is when the thumb is touched to each finger of the same hand.

19.   (1) This is unsafe; the patient cannot see and should not lead.

* (2) This allows the nurse to guide and the patient to follow; it supports comfort and contributes to confidence.

   (3) This is the method used to assist a patient with a walker who has a mobility deficit.

   (4) Corridor rails are not continuous; this method does not inspire confidence and is not as safe as option 2.

20.   (1) Reducing pressure prevents decubitus ulcers, not range of motion; range of motion prevents contractures.

* (2) Regularly extending and flexing a joint prevent permanent muscle shortening and lengthening which in turn prevent contractures.

   (3) This increases respirations and conditions the heart; aerobic conditioning is not done to increase joint range.

   (4) It increases muscle tone, not muscle size.

21.   (1) The patient has only slight hemiparesis; it is not unsafe to have both rails down as long as the nurse is at the bedside.

  * (2) This is essential because it prevents the bed or wheelchair from moving out from under the patient during transfer which could cause a fall.

    (3) This is not necessary if all safety principles are followed.

    (4) This does not provide for safety; it provides for privacy.

22.   (1) This prevents planter flexion, not external rotation.

    (2) This keeps linen off the feet and legs; it supports comfort and does not prevent external rotation.

  * (3) This prevents the hip and leg from externally rotating by positioning the leg in normal alignment.

    (4) These do not prevent external rotation; they are used to increase venous return in the lower legs.

23.   * (1) A patient using a reclining wheelchair would have minimal lower- or upper-body control; the reclining features of this wheelchair prevent a patient with poor body control from falling forward. A reclining position places excessive pressure on the sacral area; a patient with poor mobility positioned in a semi-Fowler's position would be at risk for skin breakdown due to pressure.

    (2) As long as a person can move, positioning can be changed to relieve pressure.

    (3) Same as #2.

    (4) Same as #2.

24.   * (1) This is the correct term to describe this motion.

    (2) This does not describe this action; lateral flexion is when the head is tilted as far as possible to one shoulder and then to the other shoulder.

    (3) This does not describe this action; adduction is when an extremity is moved medially and beyond if possible.

    (4) This does not describe this action; inversion is when the sole of the foot is turned medially.

25.   (1) This could contribute to feelings of dependence and loss of control.

  * (2) This supports the need to be in control; anxiety is generally reduced in proportion to an increase in control.

    (3) This is false reassurance; this denies the patient's fears.

    (4) Waiting and thinking about the transfer can increase anxiety, not reduce it; she may decide never to get out of bed.

26.   (1) They do not have a heat source; they are designed to distribute weight over the entire cushion.

  * (2) When body weight is distributed across the cushion, pressure is reduced on the tissue over bony prominences.

    (3) The body makes close contact with the cushion; air does not circulate between the patient and the cushion.

    (4) These are designed to spread body weight and reduce pressure, not limit moisture.

27.   (1) This does not put joints through their full range.

    (2) This activity will not move all joints through their normal range; prolonged sitting can cause flexion contractures of the hips and knees.

    (3) This will reduce pressure, not prevent contractures.

  * (4) Flexing and extending muscles prevents shortening or lengthening of muscles which can result in contractures.

28. * (1) This is the correct action; affected joints should be dressed first to avoid un-necessary strain. The stronger side generally has greater range.
   (2) It is unreasonable to expect self-sufficiency during the acute phase; after the acute phase the patient will have intensive rehabilitative therapy that will establish small achievable goals that will minimize frustration and support accomplishments.
   (3) Zippers are difficult to close with one hand; Velcro closures may be more appropriate.
   (4) Buttons are difficult to close with one hand; Velcro closures may be more appropriate.

29. (1) This is not the primary reason for siting on the side of the bed.
   * (2) Orthostatic hypotension is a condition that contributes to impaired stability. When moving to a sitting or standing position from lying or sitting, blood drains from the head, resulting in light-headedness and dizziness; sitting on the side of the bed allows circulation time to adjust to a change in position.
   (3) Same as #1.
   (4) Although the patient might do this, it is not the main reason for sitting on the side of the bed.

30. (1) The arms do not have to be elevated to be in normal alignment.
   (2) What is a comfortable position for the patient may not be correct alignment necessary to prevent complications; while comfort is important, functional alignment takes priority.
   * (3) Anatomical alignment maintains physical functioning, minimizes strain and stress on muscles and joints, and prevents contractures.
   (4) The head can be at the same level as the heart; it does not have to be higher.

31. (1) This absorbs moisture that keeps the skin moist which contributes to skin breakdown.
   (2) This protects the sheets from moisture, not the patient; also it generates heat because of the moisture proof backing.
   * (3) This allows air to flow through the tufts of lambs wool, helping to keep skin dry; also it reduces friction.
   (4) This reduces pressure under bony prominences, not moisture, by spreading weight over the entire mattress; it generates heat and moisture because it is generally made of plastic material.

32. (1) It is pressure that causes reduced oxygenation to local tissue, not gravity.
   * (2) This causes ischemia to local tissue. When deprived of oxygen and nutrients, pathological changes begin within 1 to 2 hours; if pressure is not relieved, tissue breakdown and cellular death occur.
   (3) Pressure causes skin breakdown.
   (4) This is a stage 4 decubitus ulcer; it is the death of tissues in response to prolonged pressure and oxygen deprivation.

33. (1) Extension is when the fingers are straightened.
   (2) Inversion refers to when the sole of the foot is turned medially.
   * (3) This is the correct term to describe the turning of the lower arm and hand so that the palm is up.
   (4) Circumduction refers to when an arm or a leg is moved in a circle.

34. (1) In this position the feet are not against the footboard; if desired a sandbag can be used to position the ankle in alignment.
     (2) This keeps linen off the feet and legs for comfort; it does not contribute to functional alignment.
  * (3) This positions the upper leg and hip in functional alignment and reduces stress and strain on the hip joint.
     (4) A pillow under the waist is used when a patient is positioned in the supine position, not the lateral position.

35. * (1) ROM can minimize or prevent the formation of joint contractures by preventing the permanent shortening of muscles, ligaments, and tendons from disuse.
     (2) This is caused by pressure, not lack of ROM.
     (3) This is caused by immobility; ROM does not prevent decreased muscle mass, endurance, or atrophy.
     (4) ROM is not done to prevent muscle spasms. Various active exercises can strengthen muscles which may prevent muscle spasm; however, passive ROM is not one of these exercises.

36. (1) This requires a physician's order.
     (2) This distributes pressure and minimizes the formation of decubitus ulcers, not contractures.
     (3) This prevents pressure that can precipitate the formation of decubitus ulcers, not contractures.
  * (4) Functional alignment is the correct geometric arrangement of body parts in relation to each other; balance is achieved without undue strain on joints, muscles, tendons, or ligaments. The muscles are usually in a slight state of tension that requires minimal muscular force yet supports the internal framework and organs.

MEETING PATIENTS' ELIMINATION NEEDS

This section encompasses questions related to bowel and bladder needs. Topics associated with intestinal elimination include incontinence, constipation, diarrhea, enemas, bowel retraining, rectal tubes, and medications. Questions also focus on needs associated with urinary elimination and include topics such as incontinence, bladder retraining, toileting, and external and internal urinary catheters.

Questions

1. To promote a successful bladder-training program, the most important nursing intervention would be:
   (1) Offering the patient a full liquid diet
   (2) Following the scheduled program exactly
   (3) Maintaining a strict intake and output record
   (4) Washing the patient's perineal area every shift

2. To help maintain continence in a patient who has urge incontinence, the nurse should:
   (1) Toilet him every 2 hours
   (2) Encourage him to stay in his room
   (3) Toilet him immediately upon request
   (4) Limit his fluid intake during the night

3. When a resident has an indwelling urinary catheter (Foley catheter), the collection bag should be:
   (1) Carried at waist level when ambulating
   (2) Kept below the level of the pelvis
   (3) Changed at least once a week
   (4) Clamped when out of bed

4. All of the following actions could be included in bladder-retraining programs. The action that would be included in *every* bladder-retraining program would be:
   (1) Providing 3000 ml of fluids a day
   (2) Toileting the patient prior to sleep
   (3) Toileting the patient every 2 hours
   (4) Utilizing adult incontinence underwear

5. When changing a condom catheter (external catheter) for an uncircumcised patient, the nurse must:
   (1) Replace the foreskin over the glans
   (2) Secure the condom directly behind the glans
   (3) Position excess tubing in loops below the bed
   (4) Apply lubricating ointment on the shaft of the penis

6. Mrs. Cardone complains about being constipated. The nurse should encourage her to ingest:
   (1) Baked chicken
   (2) Plain yogurt
   (3) Fresh fruit
   (4) White bread

7. To ambulate a patient with an indwelling urinary catheter (Foley), the nurse should:
   (1) Hang the collection bag below the patient's hips
   (2) Maintain multiple dependent loops in the tubing
   (3) Clamp the urinary tube before ambulating
   (4) Detach the tube from the collection bag

8. Women have a higher incidence of urinary tract infections than men have because:
   (1) Urine flows toward the rectum via gravity when voiding
   (2) Women must sit rather than stand when toileting
   (3) Women use bedpans which harbor microorganisms
   (4) The rectum is closer to the urinary meatus

9. Which of the following actions comes *first* in a bladder-retraining program?
   (1) Offer to toilet the patient every 2 hours.
   (2) Design an individual schedule for toileting.
   (3) Provide adequate fluids during the retraining period.
   (4) Assess the patient's ability to cooperate with the program.

10. When giving a tap water enema, the nurse recognizes that its primary purpose is to:
    (1) Minimize intestinal gas
    (2) Cleanse the bowel of stool
    (3) Reduce abdominal distension
    (4) Decrease the loss of electrolytes

11. A confused patient asks to use the bathroom even though she urinated only 30 minutes ago. The nurse should:
    (1) Take her to the bathroom and toilet the patient
    (2) Remind her that she urinated just 30 minutes ago
    (3) Request a physician's order for a Foley catheter
    (4) Persuade her to try to hold it for at least 1 hour

12. A patient on a bladder-retraining program is incontinent at 1:00 A.M. every morning. To promote continence, the nurse should plan to:
    (1) Apply an incontinence pad at bedtime
    (2) Limit the intake of fluid after dinner
    (3) Position the call bell within easy reach
    (4) Toilet the patient at 12:30 A.M. every night

13. The physician orders a 750-ml tap water enema. To best promote acceptance of the volume ordered, the nurse should:
    (1) Place the patient in the left lateral position
    (2) Have the patient take shallow breaths
    (3) Keep the fluid at body temperature
    (4) Administer the fluid slowly

14. Which of the following patients would be at the highest risk for developing diarrhea?
    (1) A child who is physically active
    (2) An elderly man who drinks a lot of fluid
    (3) A middle-age woman who eats whole-grain cereal
    (4) An adolescent who is experiencing problems in school

15. Foods likely to cause constipation are:
    (1) Fruits
    (2) Vegetables
    (3) Whole grains
    (4) Dairy products

16. Which of the following would be most effective for a patient who is unable to tolerate a large amount of enema fluid?
    (1) Hypertonic fluid
    (2) Normal saline
    (3) Soapy water
    (4) Tap water

17. Which of the following patients is at greatest risk for developing constipation?
    (1) Toddler
    (2) Adolescent
    (3) Pregnant woman
    (4) Middle-aged man

18. To best facilitate the expelling of urine from the bladder, the patient should be taught:
    (1) Pelvic floor contractions
    (2) The Valsalva maneuver
    (3) Crede compression
    (4) Kegel exercises

19. What normal physiological function of the body helps prevent infection?
    (1) Elevated temperature
    (2) High pH of gastric secretions
    (3) Flushing action of urine flow
    (4) Rapid peristalsis in the large intestine

20. When preparing a soapsuds enema for an adult, how much fluid should the nurse use?
    (1) 250 ml
    (2) 500 ml
    (3) 750 ml
    (4) 1000 ml

21. The nurse understands that diarrhea causes skin irritation mainly because it consists of:
    (1) Bile
    (2) Fiber
    (3) Fluid
    (4) Enzymes

22. Which of the following cathartics acts as a stool softener and is most effective in preventing straining during defecation?
    (1) Colace
    (2) Ducolax
    (3) Mineral oil
    (4) Milk of Magnesia

23. To promote intestinal peristalsis, a patient should be encouraged to:
    (1) Use a bulk cathartic weekly
    (2) Take caster oil once a month
    (3) Eat whole-grain foods every day
    (4) Attempt defecation at least four times a day

24. When administering an enema, the nurse should position the patient in the:
    (1) Dorsal recumbent position
    (2) Right lateral position
    (3) Back-lying position
    (4) Left Sim's position

25. When caring for a patient's elimination needs, which of the following concepts impacts on planning care?
    (1) Emotional stress decreases peristalsis.
    (2) Peristalsis increases after ingesting food.
    (3) Straining during defecation increases the heart rate.
    (4) Enema solutions should be administered at room temperature.

26. While sitting on a toilet, a person leans forward when attempting to defecate. Leaning forward specifically promotes fecal elimination because it:
    (1) Raises intra-abdominal pressure
    (2) Uses gravity to facilitate elimination
    (3) Elongates the curves of the sigmoid colon
    (4) Relaxes the internal and external rectal sphincters

27. When voiding, the male patient on bed rest should be positioned in the:
    (1) Supine position
    (2) Lateral position
    (3) Contour position
    (4) Standing position

28. In the morning a patient has a loose watery stool. To determine if the patient has diarrhea, the nurse should ask:
    (1) "When was the last time you had a similar stool?"
    (2) "Have you been drinking a lot of fluid lately?"
    (3) "Are you experiencing any abdominal cramping?"
    (4) "What did you have for dinner last night?"

29. The nurse recognizes that a rectal tube is used to:
    (1) Administer an enema
    (2) Dilate the rectal sphincter
    (3) Relieve abdominal distention
    (4) Visualize the intestinal mucosa

30. When administering a soapsuds enema, the nurse understands the primary action of the soapsuds is to:
    (1) Lower the surface tension of water
    (2) Distend the lumen of the bowel
    (3) Irritate the bowel mucosa
    (4) Exert an osmotic effect

31. Which of the following is the safest form of a laxative?
    (1) Softening agent
    (2) Osmotic cathartic
    (3) Bulk-forming agent
    (4) Stimulant cathartic

Rationales

1. (1) This is unnecessary; any kind of diet plus adequate fluid is all that is necessary.
  * (2) Toileting times are purposely scheduled in response to times of fluid intake and the patient's normal elimination pattern; to increase success, the schedule must be followed exactly.
    (3) Intake and output is unnecessary; it is not the volume of fluids and/or urine that is of interest but the pattern of voiding relative to fluid intake that is important.
    (4) Although important, this will not contribute to a patient's ability to regain continence.

2. (1) This is unnecessary; only when the patient feels the need to void does he need to be immediately toileted.
    (2) This promotes isolation and should be avoided.
  * (3) This supports continence because the person with urge incontinence must immediately void or lose control.
    (4) This may be part of a toileting program to provide for uninterrupted sleep; however, it does not address the patient's need when he has the immediate urge to void.

3. (1) This is too high; it allows urine to flow back into the bladder which can cause a urinary tract infection.
  * (2) This prevents urine from flowing back into the bladder; urine flows away from the bladder by gravity.
    (3) Collection bags are attached to a Foley and should not be disconnected; a Foley and bag should only be changed every 4 to 6 weeks unless crusting or sediment collects on the inside of the tubing.
    (4) This is unnecessary; this is unsafe for some patients.

4. (1) The volume of scheduled fluid intake is based on the individual needs of the patient.
  * (2) All patients on bladder-retraining programs are toileted prior to sleep; this contributes to less urine volume in the bladder during the night.
    (3) Toileting is not automatically implemented every 2 hours but is based on the individual needs of the patient.
    (4) Incontinence pads are generally not encouraged when implementing a retraining program; however, devices used depend on the individual needs and preferences of the patient.

5. * (1) Perineal care should be provided when changing a condom catheter; in the uncircumcised male, if the foreskin is not replaced to the normal position, it can tighten around the shaft of the penis causing local edema and pain.
   (2) This device should be secured farther up the shaft of the penis, not immediately behind the glans.
   (3) Loops should not be kept in the dependent position; dependent loops allow urine to collect, stagnate, and backup into the bladder.
   (4) The shaft of the penis should be dry; this could prevent the condom device from securely staying in place.

6. (1) Chicken does not contain roughage.
   (2) Plain yogurt contains yeast, not roughage.
   * (3) Fresh fruit contains roughage which adds bulk to stool, increasing peristalsis.
   (4) White bread does not contain roughage; the whole grain has been removed during processing.

7. * (1) This prevents the reflux of urine back up the tubing into the bladder.
   (2) Loops of tubing should not be in a dependent position; dependent loops can cause urine to collect, stagnate, and back up into the bladder.
   (3) This is unnecessary; this can be unsafe for patients recovering from surgery of the bladder.
   (4) Urinary drainage systems should always remain closed; closed systems reduce infection by preventing pathogens from entering the system.

8. (1) Urine that flows toward the rectum rarely causes infection; however, bacteria from the rectal area can cause urinary tract infections.
   (2) This should not increase the prevalence of infection.
   (3) If properly cleaned after use, bedpans are not a source of infection.
   * (4) Stool wiped toward the urinary meatus can cause urinary tract infections; *E. coli,* a common bacteria in stool, causes urinary tract infections.

9. (1) Toileting times are not automatically every 2 hours; they are individually designed based on the patient's voiding pattern and fluid intake.
   (2) This would be the second step once it is determined that the patient is motivated and able to participate and cooperate with the program.
   (3) These are interventions; first the nurse must assess the patient's ability to participate and cooperate with the program.
   * (4) This is the initial step in a bladder-retraining program. The patient must be an active participant in a bowel- or bladder-retraining program; a patient's cooperation is an essential component of a successful program.

10. (1) A Harris drip (Harris flush) helps evacuate intestinal gas, not stool.
    * (2) This introduces fluid into the intestinal tract; pressure and irritation of the intestinal mucosa increase peristalsis and evacuation of stool.
    (3) The main purpose of a tap water enema is to irritate and distend the bowel to stimulate evacuation of stool; however, a secondary gain is that it can reduce abdominal distension as flatus and stool are evacuated along with the enema solution.
    (4) This would increase the loss of electrolytes because it is a hypotonic solution.

11. * (1) This meets the patient's need to void and promotes continence; the nurse should not assume that the patient is confused or forgetful.
    (2) This denies the patient's need to void.

(3) Foley catheters should not be used to avoid incontinence or the inconvenience of frequently toileting a patient.

(4) The patient has a need to void now; an hour is too long a time period to postpone urination.

12. (1) This holds moisture against the skin which can contribute to skin breakdown; this should be avoided.

(2) This will decrease the volume of urine voided, not prevent incontinence.

(3) The patient may not have time to communicate the need to void or may be unaware of the need to void before being incontinent.

* (4) This provides the patient the opportunity to void prior to becoming incontinent; if effective, it will contribute to self-esteem and personal hygiene.

13. (1) In the left lateral position the sigmoid colon is below the rectum, facilitating the instillation of fluid; however, to best promote the acceptance of the volume ordered, the nurse should administer the fluid slowly.

(2) Deep breaths help prevent patients from holding their breath which increases intra-abdominal pressure; increased intra-abdominal pressure can interfere with the instillation and retention of enema fluid.

(3) Enema water temperature should be between 105 and 110°F; warm fluid promotes muscle relaxation and comfort. Enema fluid below 98.6°F can contribute to intestinal muscle spasm and discomfort.

* (4) Slow administration of enema fluid minimizes the probability of intestinal spasm and premature evacuation of the enema fluid before a therapeutic effect is achieved.

14. (1) Physical activity, fluid, and fiber help to prevent constipation, not precipitate diarrhea.

(2) Same as #1.

(3) Same as #1.

* (4) Psychological stress increases intestinal motility and mucus secretion, promoting diarrhea.

15. (1) These foods provide bulk (undigested residue) in the diet which facilitates fecal elimination, not constipation.

(2) Same as #1.

(3) Same as #1.

* (4) Dairy products are low in roughage and lack bulk. Dairy products produce too little waste to stimulate the defecation reflex; low-residue foods move more slowly through the intestinal tract, permitting increased fluid uptake from stool, resulting in hard-formed stools and constipation.

16. * (1) A hypertonic enema solution uses only 120 to 180 ml of solution. Hypertonic solutions expend osmotic pressure that draws fluid out of the interstitial spaces; fluid pulled into the colon and rectum distend the bowel causing an increase in peristalsis resulting in bowel evacuation.

(2) A normal saline enema is isotonic and requires a volume of 500 ml to be effective; the volume of fluid, not its saline content, causes an increase in peristalsis and evacuation of the bowel.

(3) A soapsuds enema requires a volume of 1000 to 1200 ml of fluid to result in an effective evacuation of the bowel.

(4) A tap water enema usually requires 750 ml, which is a large volume of fluid.

17.   (1) A toddler usually drinks adequate fluids, eats a regular diet, and is very active; these activities contribute to normal bowel elimination, not the development of constipation.

   (2) The adolescent usually eats more food than he or she did at earlier stages and may complain of indigestion, not constipation; indigestion is a response to increased gastric acidity that occurs during adolescence.

   * (3) The growing size of the fetus exerts pressure on the rectum and bowel which causes some obstruction of the intestines, contributing to constipation; the decreased motility causes increased absorption of water, promoting constipation.

   (4) This age is at risk for weight gain due to a decrease in activity and metabolism, not constipation.

18.   (1) Pelvic floor exercises help to enable a person to start and stop a stream of urine. These exercises include trying to stop and start the stream of urine while urinating; they also include the contraction and relaxation of the anterior and posterior muscles of the pelvic floor while in a sitting or standing position. Pelvic floor exercises are done to improve one's ability to retain urine, not pass urine.

   (2) This increases the intra-abdominal pressure in an effort to expel stool; this is accomplished when people hold their breath during a forced expiration and contract the abdominal muscles. The levator ani muscle relaxes and permits feces to be expelled.

   * (3) The Crede method stimulates micturition and relaxation of the urethral sphincter via external manual compression of the bladder.

   (4) This is isometric exercising of the pubococcygeal muscle which is the muscle associated with the urinary sphincter; this improves one's ability to retain urine, not pass urine.

19.   (1) An elevated temperature results from released toxins in the presence of infection; it may help to limit an already existing infection, but it will not prevent an infection.

   (2) Gastric secretions are acidic and have a low pH.

   * (3) Microorganisms congregate at the urinary meatus because it is warm, moist, and dark; when urine flows down the urethra and out the urinary meatus, the force of the urine carries microorganisms away which prevents ascending infections.

   (4) Rapid peristalsis results in diarrhea; this is not a normal physiological function.

20.   (1) This is too little fluid to administer to an adult to stimulate effective evacuation of the bowel when administering a soapsuds enema; this is the recommended amount the nurse might administer to a toddler. Hypertonic solutions only need 120 to 180 ml of solution to achieve effective results, not a soapsuds enema.

   (2) This is too little fluid to stimulate effective evacuation of the bowel when administering a soapsuds enema to an adult; this is the recommended amount of solution the nurse might administer to a large school-age child or small adolescent.

(3) This is too little fluid to stimulate effective evacuation of the bowel when administering a soapsuds enema to an adult. This is the recommended amount of solution the nurse might administer to an average-sized adolescent; this is also the amount of volume suggested for saline and tap water enemas.

* (4) This is the average suggested volume of soapsuds solution administered to an adult to stimulate effective evacuation of the bowel; it provides enough fluid to fill the bowel and apply pressure to the intestinal mucosa to stimulate defecation.

21. (1) Although irritating, bile is not as caustic as digestive enzymes. The components of bile include bilirubin, bile salts, cholesterol, lecithin, fatty acids, electrolytes, and water. Bile salts are the components that are metabolically active; bile salts increase fat solubility which enables fat to pass through the intestinal wall.

(2) Fiber is bulk that distends the lumen of the bowel and by itself does not irritate the skin.

(3) Although fluid on the skin contributes to tissue irritation, it is the enzymes in feces that erode the skin.

* (4) Enzymes are biologic catalysts that speed up chemical reactions; digestive enzymes break down nutrient cells by hydrolysis and therefore are also extremely caustic to the skin.

22. * (1) Dioctyl sodium sulfosuccinate (Colace) is a detergent that lowers the surface tension of feces, allowing penetration by water and fat which soften stool.

(2) Bisacodyl is a stimulant and cathartic because it irritates the intestinal mucosa, increasing intestinal motility.

(3) Mineral oil is a lubricant that softens the fecal mass; regular use interferes with the absorption of fat-soluble vitamins A, D, E, and K.

(4) Magnesium hydroxide (Milk of Magnesia) is a saline or osmotic agent that draws water into the fecal mass.

23. (1) Routine intake of cathartics should be avoided to prevent dependence.

(2) Same as #1.

* (3) Whole grains provide fiber and bulk which distend the bowel lumen promoting intestinal peristalsis.

(4) Frequent excessive straining at stool can precipitate hemorrhoids. Intestinal peristalsis is usually increased 1 hour after meals because of the gastrocolic reflex; attempting defecation after meals increases the chances of evacuating the bowel.

24. (1) This position would not utilize the natural curve of the rectum and sigmoid colon to facilitate instillation of the enema solution.

(2) Same as #1.

(3) Same as #1.

* (4) This permits solution to flow downward by gravity along the natural curve of the rectum and sigmoid colon, promoting instillation and retention of the solution.

25. (1) Emotional stress usually increases peristalsis.

* (2) Food or fluid that enters and fills the stomach or the duodenum stimulates peristalsis; this is called the "gastrocolic reflex" or "duodenocolic reflex."

(3) Straining at defecation does not increase the heart rate; the Valsalva maneuver raises the intrathoracic pressure which impedes venous return and ever so slightly decreases the heart rate.

(4) Enema solutions should be administered slightly above body temperature (105 to 110°F).

26. * (1) When a person leans forward while in the sitting position, intra-abdominal pressure increases, facilitating fecal elimination.

(2) The sitting position utilizes gravity to facilitate defecation, not leaning forward.

(3) When sitting and leaning forward, the curves of the sigmoid colon remain unchanged.

(4) Relaxation of the internal and external rectal sphincters may result in response to this position; however, this relaxation of sphincters is in response to increased intra-abdominal pressure.

27. (1) This position would not promote passage of urine through the urinary tract via gravity.

* (2) This position is the closest to the normal standing position used by men to void; the hips and knees are almost extended, and the hands can be used for self-care.

(3) In this position the hips and knees are flexed and the perineal area is dependent in relation to the knees; placing and using a urinal in this position without spilling would be difficult.

(4) This is contraindicated because the patient is not allowed out of bed.

28. * (1) Diarrhea is the defecation of liquid feces and increased frequency of defecation; there should be more than one episode to be considered diarrhea.

(2) Excessive fluid intake is excreted through the kidneys, not the intestinal tract.

(3) Cramping is not specific to diarrhea; it can also be associated with constipation and intestinal obstruction.

(4) While this answer may help determine if food influenced the patient's intestinal elimination, it will not further assess the presence of diarrhea.

29. (1) An enema tube is used to administer an enema; a rectal tube is different and is used to provide temporary relief from flatulence.

(2) This is not the purpose of a rectal tube.

* (3) A rectal tube is inserted past the anal sphincters (6 inches in an adult and 2 to 4 inches in a child) and left in place for 30-minute intervals every 2 to 3 hours. Rectal tubes are used to promote the passage of flatus, reducing abdominal distention.

(4) A rectal tube is not designed to visualize the intestinal mucosa. A proctoscope is an instrument designed to visualize the rectum, a sigmoidoscope is an instrument designed to visualize the sigmoid colon and the rectum, and a colonoscope is an instrument designed to visualize the entire large intestine.

30. (1) This is the rationale for using soap when administering a bed bath.

(2) This is the rationale for using a particular volume of fluid.

* (3) Soap is an irritant that stimulates the intestinal mucosa, precipitating peristalsis and the eventual evacuation of stool.

(4) This is the rationale for using a hypertonic solution, not soapsuds.

31.   (1) Softening agents reduce the surface tension of feces through detergent action; softening agents allow feces to absorb water and fat, causing stool to become large, soft, and easy to defecate.
       (2) Osmotic cathartics draw water into the fecal mass via osmotic action; the body attempts to dilute the salt preparation in the cathartic by pulling water, causing lubrication and increased bulk of stool.
   * (3) Bulk-forming agents absorb water and increase intestinal bulk. Bulk stretches the intestinal walls stimulating peristalsis; bulk-forming agents are the least irritating and therefore the safest cathartic.
       (4) Stimulant cathartics cause local irritation to the intestinal mucosa; they also minimize absorption of water in the large intestines. Stimulant cathartics are more caustic than bulk-forming agents in stimulating peristalsis.

MEETING PATIENTS' OXYGEN NEEDS

This section encompasses questions related to assessments and interventions associated with normal and abnormal respiratory and circulatory function. Questions focus on topics such as preventing aspiration, providing emergency care for aspiration, techniques and devices that assess or increase respiratory or circulatory function, and assessments and interventions associated with the administration of oxygen.

Questions

1. The nurse must provide physical hygiene to a patient receiving a nasogastric tube feeding. To prevent aspiration while administering care, the nurse should:
   (1) Shut the feeding off
   (2) Slow the rate of flow
   (3) Seek additional assistance
   (4) Lower the height of the bag

2. A patient walking in the hall complains of sudden chest pain. The initial intervention by the nurse should be to:
   (1) Take the patient's vital signs
   (2) Perform a detailed pain assessment
   (3) Walk the patient back to her room slowly
   (4) Get a chair so the patient can sit and rest

3. When oxygen therapy via nasal cannula is ordered for a patient, the *first* action by the nurse is to:
   (1) Lubricate the nares with water-soluble jelly
   (2) Explain the rules of fire safety and oxygen use
   (3) Adjust the oxygen level before applying the cannula
   (4) Post an "oxygen in use" sign on the door to the room

4. To prevent aspiration after meals by a patient who has difficulty swallowing, the nurse should *first:*
   (1) Position the patient in the low-Fowler's position
   (2) Provide a pitcher of water at the bedside
   (3) Encourage mouth care when necessary
   (4) Inspect the mouth for pocketed food

5. When a patient chokes on food and is unable to speak, the nurse should first:
   (1) Clap between the scapulae three times
   (2) Initiate the abdominal thrust maneuver

(3) Instruct the patient to swallow forcefully
(4) Begin rescue breathing within 4 minutes

6. A patient with a history of respiratory disease begins to have difficulty breathing. The assessment that would indicate the most serious complication would be:
   (1) Wheezing sounds on inspiration
   (2) Mucus tinged with franc red streaks
   (3) Orthostatic hypotension when rising
   (4) The need to sit in the orthopneic position

7. The MOST important intervention by the nurse to increase both circulation and respiration in a patient is to:
   (1) Encourage the use of a spirometer
   (2) Massage bony prominences with lotion
   (3) Reposition the patient every 2 hours
   (4) Teach the patient to cough and deep breath

8. A patient who is short of breath is receiving oxygen through a nasal cannula. To prevent skin breakdown around the nares, the nurse should:
   (1) Remove the tubing for 15 minutes every 2 hours
   (2) Turn and position the patient every 2 hours
   (3) Adjust the cannula so it is comfortable
   (4) Provide oral hygiene whenever necessary

9. While eating, Mr. Dole clutches his upper chest with his hands, appears unable to breathe, and has a frightened facial expression. The most appropriate initial action by the nurse is to:
   (1) Perform the abdominal thrust maneuver
   (2) Start artificial respirations
   (3) Slap him three times on the back
   (4) Ask him if he can speak

10. All of the following are observed by the nurse when giving mouth care to an unconscious patient. The assessment that requires immediate intervention is:
    (1) Saliva drooling out of the mouth
    (2) A gurgling sound when breathing
    (3) Sordes found on the hard palate
    (4) Lesions on the gingival tissue

11. The most appropriate site of the body to assess for the presence of cyanosis is the:
    (1) Face
    (2) Lower legs
    (3) Fingernail beds
    (4) Conjunctiva of the eyes

12. To reduce anxiety related to the use of oxygen via nasal cannula, the nurse should say:
    (1) "Keep calm and everything will be OK."
    (2) "This is oxygen; it will help your breathing."
    (3) "This is a treatment that was ordered by your doctor."
    (4) "This oxygen will be discontinued as soon as possible."

13. Mrs. Debow has difficulty swallowing her food. To prevent her from aspirating when eating, the nurse should:
    (1) Promote a conversation during meals for socialization
    (2) Encourage her to drink fluid before swallowing food
    (3) Allow enough time between spoonfuls for chewing
    (4) Cut up the meat and mix it with the soft food

14. During the night a patient complains of being short of breath. The nurse's initial action should be to:
    (1) Obtain vital signs
    (2) Raise the head of the bed
    (3) Administer emergency oxygen
    (4) Encourage pursed-lip breathing

15. When a patient has prolonged impaired peripheral arterial circulation, the nurse should assess for:
    (1) Cyanosis
    (2) Tachycardia
    (3) Yellow toenails
    (4) Continuous leg discomfort

16. When implementing chest physiotherapy, the nurse teaches the patient that the primary purpose is to:
    (1) Alter the tracheobronchial mucosa
    (2) Change the consistency of sputum
    (3) Mobilize secretion
    (4) Induce coughing

17. When monitoring a patient's status through pulse oximetry, the nurse is assessing the patient's:
    (1) Heart rate
    (2) Vital signs
    (3) Blood pressure
    (4) Oxygen saturation

18. Which of the following individuals would most likely have life-threatening complications when experiencing a respiratory infection?
    (1) Infant
    (2) Adolescent
    (3) Elderly person
    (4) School-age child

19. When assessing Mr. Singers's breath sounds, the nurse identifies wheezing. The nurse recognizes that this occurs when:
    (1) There is fluid in the lung
    (2) Air moves through a narrowed airway
    (3) The patient sits in the orthopneic position
    (4) The pleural sack rubs against the lung surface

20. A patient receiving oxygen by nasal cannula has an elevation of the clavicles on inspiration. When planning care, which of the following interventions should take priority?
    (1) Pace care
    (2) Promote bed rest
    (3) Increase the O_2 flow rate
    (4) Monitor respiratory rate every hour

21. Kussmaul respirations are characterized by:
    (1) Abnormally deep, rapid inhalations
    (2) An excessive effort to inhale and exhale
    (3) A rate of breathing that is slow and regular
    (4) Alternating periods of apnea and deep, rapid breathing

22. Which of the following individuals would have the most dramatic increase in the need for oxygen?
    (1) A pregnant woman
    (2) A man with a fever

(3) A person exercising

(4) A patient under anesthesia

23. To BEST evaluate peripheral circulation in a lower extremity, the nurse should assess the:
    (1) Capillary refill in the toenails
    (2) Blood pressure in the extremity
    (3) Presence of hair on the toes
    (4) Color of the foot

24. The nurse assesses that the patient understands diaphragmatic breathing when the patient says, "I should:
    (1) Feel my abdomen flatten on inspiration."
    (2) Raise my shoulders and chest when I inhale."
    (3) Hold my breath for 3 seconds on inspiration."
    (4) Place my palms against the abdomen when I inhale."

25. Which of the following is most effective for maintaining a patent airway?
    (1) Active coughing
    (2) Abdominal breathing
    (3) Incentive spirometry
    (4) Nebulizer treatments

26. A patient has anemia which has compromised the ability to meet the body's oxygen needs. The nurse recognizes that this oxygen problem is related to the inability to:
    (1) Transport oxygen
    (2) Exchange oxygen
    (3) Perfuse oxygen
    (4) Diffuse oxygen

27. A common local adaptation to pressure is specifically referred to as:
    (1) Edema
    (2) Ischemia
    (3) Orthopnea
    (4) Hypovolemia

28. When inserting an oral airway, the initial action of the nurse is to:
    (1) Insert it with the curve toward the tongue
    (2) Lightly lubricate the airway with Vaseline
    (3) Ensure that the airway is the correct size
    (4) Sweep the oral cavity with a gloved finger

29. The adequacy of tissue oxygenation is most accurately measured by:
    (1) Hemoglobin levels
    (2) Hematocrit values
    (3) Arterial blood gases
    (4) Pulmonary function tests

30. The nurse assesses a patient's breathing and identifies that the pattern is alternating between apnea and deep rapid breathing. When documenting this assessment, the nurse writes that the patient's respiratory pattern reflects:
    (1) Kussmaul respirations
    (2) Apneustic respirations
    (3) Paradoxical respirations
    (4) Cheyne-Stokes respirations

31. The nurse recognizes that the work of normal breathing is based on the:
    (1) Competence of the phrenic nerve to innervate accessory muscles
    (2) Ability of the intrapleural pressure to become positive

(3) Capability of the diaphragm to fall during expiration
(4) Lack of resistance in the airway during inspiration

32. When applying a pulse oximetry sensor to the patient's finger, the nurse should:
    (1) Remove frosted nail polish from the patient's nails
    (2) Send the patient's rings home with a family member
    (3) Keep the hand continuously elevated on a pillow
    (4) Shave any hair that might be on the finger

33. Which of the following patients with a respiratory tract infection would have the highest risk for an airway obstruction?
    (1) 2-year-old toddler
    (2) 16-year-old child
    (3) Middle-aged woman
    (4) Elderly man

34. A productive cough means it:
    (1) Precipitates pain
    (2) Results in sputum
    (3) Gets progressively worse
    (4) Interferes with breathing

35. The nurse recognizes that a fever can result in tachypnea because of the:
    (1) Need to retain carbon dioxide
    (2) Increase in the metabolic rate
    (3) Decrease in carbon dioxide levels
    (4) Attempt to compensate for respiratory alkalosis

36. The nurse recognizes that the exchange of respiratory gases is based on the principle of:
    (1) Osmosis
    (2) Invasion
    (3) Diffusion
    (4) Decompression

37. When implementing nasotracheal suctioning in an adult, the nurse:
    (1) Uses wall suction with a pressure setting below 90 mm Hg
    (2) Applies intermittent suction during removal of the catheter
    (3) Employs a rotating motion during insertion of the catheter
    (4) Suctions the nasotracheal area after the oropharyngeal area

Rationales

1. * (1) This reduces the risk of aspiration by temporarily halting the administration of an additional volume of feeding.
    (2) It needs to be shut off, not just slowed, to reduce the risk of aspiration by temporarily halting the administration of an additional volume of feeding.
    (3) This will not reduce the risk of aspiration; the feeding should be temporarily halted.
    (4) This will only slow the rate of the feeding, not halt its flow.

2. (1) The patient needs to rest the heart; this action will delay meeting this need. Vital signs can be taken once the patient is resting.
    (2) This can be done once the patient is resting.

(3) This should be avoided; activity increases the demand on the heart and will increase the pain.

* (4) Reducing activity decreases the oxygen demand on the heart; this will in turn reduce the pain.

3. (1) This is not necessary; nares should only be cleaned with soap and water daily and when necessary.

* (2) Safety is a priority; patients must understand the rules related to oxygen use and that oxygen supports combustion.

(3) This is done after explaining the procedure.

(4) Same as #3.

4. (1) A high-Fowler's position facilitates retention by gravity.

(2) Fluids can be easily aspirated by a patient who has difficulty swallowing; fluid intake should be supervised.

(3) Frequent mouth care will provide comfort, but it will not reduce the risk of aspiration unless pocketed food is removed.

* (4) This is an important action; patients who have difficulty swallowing do not recognize that food can become trapped and pocketed on the weak side of the mouth.

5. (1) This could cause aspirated food to lodge deeper in the respiratory passages.

* (2) This maneuver pushes trapped air out of the lungs, forcing out the obstructing food.

(3) This will not clear the airway. Air needs to be forced out of the lungs; attempting to swallow could cause further aspiration.

(4) This could force the obstruction deeper into the breathing passages; the nurse first needs to implement the Heimlich maneuver.

6. (1) This is a common response by individuals with chronic respiratory disease; elevating the head helps breathing by lowering the abdominal organs by gravity which allows the diaphragm to contract more efficiently on inspiration.

* (2) This is not a common response to chronic respiratory disease and should be reported immediately.

(3) Same as #1.

(4) This is not uncommon for patients with chronic respiratory disease; however, if it progresses, it should be reported immediately.

7. (1) This only helps to prevent respiratory complications.

(2) This only increases local circulation.

* (3) This prevents fluid from collecting in lung fields which can cause infection, thereby promoting respirations; it relieves pressure and increases activity, thereby promoting circulation.

(4) Same as #1.

8. (1) This is too long a period of time to remove oxygen for a patient in need of oxygen.

(2) This prevents pressure ulcers of the body but will not prevent skin breakdown around the nares.

* (3) If the cannula comfortably rests in the nostrils, it will avoid pressure on the nares that can cause skin breakdown.

(4) While adequate oral hygiene is important, it is mainly pressure that causes skin breakdown; oral hygiene alone does not prevent skin breakdown.

9.   (1) This is done once it is determined that the patient cannot speak.

      (2) The patient is not in respiratory arrest; he has food lodged in the respiratory passages. The initial intervention is different for each of these situations.

      (3) This could cause the aspirated object to lodge deeper in the respiratory passages.

    * (4) If the patient can speak, the airway is not totally obstructed; it is safer to allow the patient time to attempt to clear the airway by coughing.

10.   (1) This is expected; saliva should exit from the mouth and away from the airway.

    * (2) This indicates fluid or mucus in the airway; it may be necessary to suction this material out of the airway of an unconscious patient if the patient does not cough.

      (3) Although this indicates a need for more frequent mouth care, it is not an emergency.

      (4) Same as #3.

11.   (1) When experiencing a lack of oxygen, the skin of the face first will become pale before it becomes cyanotic.

      (2) The lower legs are not the first sites to assess for systemic oxygen depravation.

    * (3) Nail beds, lips, and mucous membranes of the mouth are the primary sites to assess for early signs of oxygen depravation.

      (4) Pallor of the conjunctiva of the eyes, not cyanosis, reflects reduced oxy-hemoglobin.

12.   (1) This is false reassurance; it minimizes the patient's concerns.

    * (2) This provides information and an explanation; this generally reduces fear and increases understanding and compliance.

      (3) This does not address the fact that patients have a right to know what is being done and why.

      (4) This could intensify fear if the oxygen is not discontinued; it does not provide an explanation.

13.   (1) This could increase the risk for aspiration. People should not talk with food in their mouths; people need to inhale before talking, and this action could cause aspiration of food if food is in the mouth.

      (2) This could flush food into the breathing passages rather than down the esophagus.

    * (3) Well-chewed food is broken down and mixed with saliva, forming a bolus of food; a bolus of food is easier to swallow and causes less risk of aspiration.

      (4) The patient has no difficulty chewing; food does not need to be cut up as long as the patient has the time to adequately chew the food before attempting to swallow.

14.   (1) This action does not facilitate breathing.

    * (2) This facilitates breathing. Gravity aids the expansion of the diaphragm during inspiration; it also reduces the resistance of body weight on the chest during inspiration.

      (3) This can further compromise respiratory compensatory mechanisms if the cause of the shortness of breath is due to chronic obstructive pulmonary disease (COPD); oxygen can precipitate CO_2 narcosis in patients with COPD.

      (4) This helps patients with emphysema to exhale; diaphragmatic breathing is most effective for patients who are short of breath.

15. (1) Pallor reflects poor peripheral arterial perfusion.
  (2) This is precipitated by systemic hypoxia, not peripheral tissue hypoxia.
  * (3) This indicates prolonged tissue hypoxia; there is a decrease in oxygen and nutrients to the area.
  (4) Leg discomfort related to decreased peripheral arterial perfusion is usually intermittent and associated with activity (intermittent claudication).

16. (1) Chest physiotherapy will not alter the tracheobronchial mucosa; it mobilizes secretions within the respiratory tract.
  (2) Chest physiotherapy does not change the consistency of sputum; it mobilizes sputum. An increased fluid intake will promote a less tenacious sputum.
  * (3) Chest percussion (cupping, clapping) and vibration mechanically dislodge tenacious secretions from the walls of the respiratory passages, while postural drainage drains secretions from various lung segments via gravity. Collectively these actions are called "chest physiotherapy" or "pulmonary toileting."
  (4) The mobilization of secretions may eventually induce coughing.

17. (1) When palpating a peripheral pulse or auscultating the apical rate, the nurse obtains the heart rate.
  (2) Vital signs are temperature, pulse, respirations, and blood pressure, not oxygen saturation.
  (3) Blood pressure is one of the vital signs, and it reflects the pressures exerted by the blood as it pulsates through the arteries.
  * (4) Oxygen saturation via pulse oximetry measures the degree to which hemoglobin is saturated with oxygen; it provides some indication of the efficiency of lung ventilation.

18. * (1) Infants and toddlers are at serious risk for airway obstruction which can develop as a result of respiratory tract infection; epiglottitis, bronchiolitis, and laryngospasm are acute conditions with a sudden onset that have serious implications if not immediately treated.
  (2) The healthy adolescent usually does not encounter any serious event in response to respiratory infections.
  (3) While the respiratory system undergoes changes during the aging process and there is a decline in respiratory function, complications related to infection are usually not as acute, sudden, or life threatening as with the infant.
  (4) The healthy school-age child usually does not encounter any serious event in response to respiratory infections; however, school-age children generally have respiratory infections more frequently due to exposure to other children.

19. (1) Sounds caused by fluid in the alveoli are called "rales," and sounds caused by fluid or resistance in the bronchi are called "rhonchi."
  * (2) Wheezes occur as air passes through air passages narrowed by secretions, edema, or tumors; these high-pitched squeaky musical sounds are best heard on expiration and are usually not changed by coughing.
  (3) Positioning is unrelated to adventitious sounds (abnormal breath sounds).
  (4) This is a pleural friction rub. It is a superficial grating sound heard particularly at the height of inspiration and not relieved by coughing; it is caused by rubbing together of inflamed pleural surfaces.

20. * (1) When the patient uses accessory muscles to increase lung volume during inspiration, the work of breathing increases. This places greater demands on the body to increase the metabolic rate which increases the need for oxygen; pacing care allows for rest which reduces the physical demand for oxygen.
   (2) Whether a patient is or is not on bed rest, care will still need to be delivered in a manner that minimizes exertion; pacing care is the priority.
   (3) Determining the oxygen flow rate is a dependent function of the nurse and requires a physician's order. In addition, too high concentrations of oxygen will diminish the respiratory drive in some people (individuals with chronic obstructive pulmonary disease) because the respiratory drive is stimulated by a decrease in oxygen in the blood, not an increase in blood carbon dioxide levels.
   (4) The respiratory rate is not the only sign that should be monitored when a patient is receiving oxygen; other changes in vital signs can occur such as increased depth and character of respirations, increased pulse rate, and elevated blood pressure. Apprehension, decreased level of consciousness, decreased ability to concentrate, behavioral changes, pallor, cyanosis, dizziness, dyspnea, and increased fatigue are also signs that indicate hypoxia.

21. * (1) Deep rapid respirations, Kussmaul respirations, is the body's effort to blow off excessive carbon dioxide, which attempts to correct metabolic acidosis.
   (2) This indicates dyspnea.
   (3) In Kussmaul respirations the breaths are rapid.
   (4) These are Cheyne-Stokes respirations; the breathing cycle begins with slow shallow breaths that gradually increase to an abnormal depth and rate, then the breaths gradually become slower and more shallow until there is a period of apnea, and then the cycle begins again.

22.   (1) A pregnant woman's metabolic rate is increased; however, pregnancy does not place as high a demand on the body's need for oxygen as exercise.
   (2) A fever causes an increase in a person's metabolic rate; however, a fever does not place as high a demand on the body's need for oxygen as exercise.
 * (3) All types of exercise dramatically increase the metabolic rate, which in turn increase the body's demand for oxygen.
   (4) General anesthesia relaxes the muscles of the body; when muscles are relaxed, the metabolic rate decreases and the demand for oxygen also decreases.

23. * (1) Applying pressure to a toenail causes blanching, and when the pressure is released, the normal color should quickly return (within 1 to 2 seconds) indicating adequate arterial perfusion.
   (2) Blood pressure reflects the pressure exerted by the blood as it pulsates through the arteries. Although people with arteriosclerosis may have increased resistance and therefore hypertension, a blood pressure does not evaluate peripheral circulation in the lower extremities as does inspection and palpation.
   (3) Although lack of hair on the feet and lower legs may indicate prolonged hypoxia, other factors such as genetic endowment may cause a lack of hair.
   (4) Assessing the color of one foot is inadequate; both feet must be assessed and compared.

24.   (1) The abdomen rises on inspiration.
   (2) These accessory muscles should not consciously be involved with diaphragmatic breathing; the abdomen should rise and fall rather than the shoulders; the chest will naturally expand and recoil.

(3) Diaphragmatic breathing involves a pattern of a slow deep inhalation followed by a slow exhalation with a tightening of the abdominal muscles to aid exhalation; the patient should not hold the breath at any time during the cycle.

* (4) This encourages the patient to feel and concentrate on the abdomen rising during inhalation and falling and contracting on exhalation.

25. * (1) A cough forcefully expels air from the lungs and is an effective self-protective reflex to clear the trachea, bronchi, and lungs of secretions.

(2) This breathing technique does not clear the air passages. It helps to decrease air trapping and reduce the work of breathing; it is used postoperatively, during labor, and with pulmonary disease to promote relaxation and pain control.

(3) This is a device used to encourage voluntary deep breathing, not to clear an airway; it is used to prevent or treat atelectasis.

(4) This does not clear an airway; it adds moisture or medication to inspired air to alter the tracheobronchial mucosa. Once the respiratory passages are dilated or mucolytic agents have reduced the viscosity of secretions, the patient can cough more productively.

26. * (1) The hemoglobin portion of red blood cells carries oxygen from the alveolar capillaries to distant tissue sites.

(2) This occurs in the capillary beds of the alveoli via the process of diffusion; this is unrelated to anemia.

(3) This relates to the extent of inflow and outflow of air between the alveoli and pulmonary capillaries, integrity of pulmonary blood vessels, or extent of blood flow to the pulmonary capillary bed. Perfusion is not related to red blood cell levels.

(4) A problem with diffusion occurs at the alveolar capillary beds and is not related to anemia.

27. (1) Edema is fluid in the interstitial compartment.

* (2) Ischemia is lack of blood supply to a body part (tissue ischemia).

(3) Orthopnea is the ability to breathe only in an upright position such as sitting or standing.

(4) Hypovolemia is a reduction in blood volume.

28. (1) This is contraindicated; this can cause the tongue to occlude the airway; the curve is rotated toward the tongue and into position after the airway has been inserted sideways along the roof of the mouth and the flange touches the mouth.

(2) A water-soluble lubricant should be used.

* (3) Adult, child, and infant sizes are available; the correct size must be used to prevent oropharnygeal trauma and promote an open airway.

(4) The nurse should avoid putting a finger into the mouth of an unconscious patient because the patient may bite down and injure the nurse; airways should be used only with an unconscious patient because in a conscious patient it stimulates the gag reflex, promoting regurgitation and aspiration.

29. (1) Although hemoglobin is the red pigment in red blood cells that carries oxygen, it is not an accurate test for adequacy of tissue oxygenation; a low hemoglobin is evidence of iron-deficiency anemia or bleeding.

(2) Although hematocrit is the percentage of red blood cell mass in proportion to whole blood, it is not an accurate test for adequacy of tissue oxygenation; a low hematocrit may indicate possible water intoxication, and an elevated hematocrit may indicate dehydration.

* (3) Arterial blood gases include the partial pressures of oxygen and carbon dioxide; they determine the adequacy of alveolar gas exchange and the ability of the lungs and kidneys to maintain the acid-base balance of body fluids.

(4) Pulmonary function tests measure lung volume and capacity; although these are valuable data they do not provide specific data about tissue oxygenation.

30. (1) Kussmaul respirations have an increase rate and depth; this is associated with metabolic acidosis and renal failure.

(2) Apneustic respirations have a prolonged gasping inspiration followed by a short, inefficient expiration; this is associated with central nervous system disorders.

(3) With paradoxical respirations the chest wall balloons on expiration and is depressed or pulled downward on inspiration; this is associated with flail chest as a result of fractured ribs.

* (4) Cheyne-Stokes breathing has a rhythmic waxing and waning of respirations. The breaths vary from very deep to very shallow followed by a brief period of apnea; this is associated with brain damage, increased intracranial pressure, and cardiac failure.

31. (1) The phrenic nerve innervates the diaphragm, not the accessory muscles.

(2) For air to flow into the lungs, the intrapleural pressure must become negative, not positive.

(3) On expiration the diaphragm rises, not falls.

* (4) Clear air passages are essential for adequate volumes of air to reach the lungs; airway resistance increases in response to an obstruction of the airway, edema of the lining of the air passages, or a disease of the respiratory passages.

32. * (1) The ingredients in acrylic nails or black, blue, green, metallic, or frosted nail polish will interfere with an accurate reading.

(2) Rings can be worn, or the reading can be taken on a finger without a ring; metal jewelry does not interfere with the reading.

(3) It is unnecessary to elevate the site being monitored; however, the pulse oximeter may identify motion as arterial pulsations. It may be necessary to immobilize, not elevate, the monitoring site to achieve accurate readings.

(4) The removal of body hair is unnecessary to achieve an accurate reading.

33. * (1) Because of the small size of the respiratory system and its narrow passages in the toddler, this age group is at risk for obstruction as a result of edema associated with the inflammatory response.

(2) Although all patients with a respiratory tract infection should be monitored for obstruction, this age group is not at as high a risk for an obstruction as a toddler.

(3) Same as #2.

(4) Same as #2.

34. (1) A productive cough may or may not produce pain depending on the patient's underlying condition.

* (2) A productive cough is accompanied by expectorated secetions.

(3) Productive does not indicate progressive.

(4) When a patient raises respiratory secretions and expectorates them, breathing usually improves.

35. (1) The body has a need to exhale carbon dioxide.
   * (2) Because of the energy required to "fight" an infection, the basal metabolic rate increases, resulting in an increased respiratory rate.
     (3) Tachypnea occurs in the presence of elevated levels of carbon dioxide and carbonic acid.
     (4) With infection the patient is more likely to be in metabolic acidosis; tachypnea that progresses to hyperventilation causes respiratory alkalosis.

36. (1) Osmosis is the passage of a solvent through a semipermeable membrane from an area of lesser solute concentration to an area of greater solute concentration.
     (2) "Invasion" refers to metastasis of a tumor by direct extension.
   * (3) Diffusion is the movement of gases from an area of greater pressure or concentration to an area of lesser pressure or concentration.
     (4) Decompression is the lowering of pressure within a space by removing fluid or gas; for example, a nasogastric tube to suction removes gastric contents decompressing the stomach.

37. (1) For wall suctioning to be effective when suctioning an adult, it should be maintained at 110 to 150 mm Hg.
   * (2) Intermittent suction is exerted on withdrawal of the suction catheter; this prevents trauma to any one section of the respiratory mucosa because of prolonged suction pressure.
     (3) The catheter is rotated on removal, not insertion of the catheter; rotating the catheter removes secretions from all surfaces of the respiratory mucosa as the catheter is withdrawn.
     (4) The opposite is acceptable technique; the nasotracheal area is considered sterile and is suctioned before the oropharyngeal area which is considered clean; this minimizes contamination of the sterile area.

ADMINISTRATION OF MEDICATIONS

This section encompasses questions related to the principles associated with the administration of medications via the oral, parenteral (intravenous piggyback and intramuscular, intradermal, and subcutaneous injections), topical, ear, eye, vaginal, and rectal routes. Questions focus on allergies, untoward effects, toxic effects, troches, developmental considerations, the Z-track method, and peak and trough levels of medications.

Questions

1. Prior to administering a medication that is teratogenic, the nurse should ask the patient:
   (1) "Have you ever had an anaphylactic reaction?"
   (2) "Were you ever addicted to drugs?"
   (3) "Do you have any allergies?"
   (4) "Are you pregnant?"

2. Which of the following statements would indicate that the patient needed further teaching regarding care of the eyes and eye medications?
   (1) "Excess medication on the eyelid can be wiped away."
   (2) "I should gaze downward while instilling the eye drops."

(3) "I should place one drop of the medication inside my lower eyelid."

(4) "The risk of transmitting infection from one eye to the other is high."

3. The nurse changes the needle after drawing up the required dosage of a caustic drug. This is done primarily because the needle is:
   (1) Too long for the required route
   (2) Coated with the medication
   (3) No longer sterile
   (4) Not as sharp

4. Besides its therapeutic effect of inhibiting microbial growth, a specific antibiotic may also depress the bone marrow. This response is classified as:
   (1) An overdose
   (2) A side-effect
   (3) A drug toxicity
   (4) An idiosyncratic effect

5. When administering a 2 ml intramuscular injection to a patient in severe pain, the site that would be most safe and therapeutic for this patient would be the:
   (1) Deltoid
   (2) Ventrogluteal
   (3) Rectus femoris
   (4) Vastus lateralis

6. A patient is to receive a medication in the form of a troche. The nurse should prepare to administer this drug via the:
   (1) Rectal route
   (2) Buccal cavity
   (3) Vaginal vault
   (4) Auditory canal

7. The nurse would recognize that the patient understood the teaching about how to self-administer a rectal suppository when the patient:
   (1) Requested sterile gloves to perform the insertion
   (2) Allowed the suppository to warm to room temperature
   (3) Held his breath during insertion of the suppository
   (4) Assumed the left-side-lying position for the insertion

8. When using an insulin syringe to administer insulin, the nurse should insert the needle at an angle of:
   (1) 30°
   (2) 45°
   (3) 90°
   (4) 180°

9. When administering oral medication to children, the MOST important factor to consider is their:
   (1) Age
   (2) Weight
   (3) Level of anxiety
   (4) Developmental level

10. When instilling ear drops into the ear of an adult, the nurse should:
    (1) Gently press a cotton ball into the ear canal
    (2) Pull the pinna of the ear downward and backward
    (3) Instill the ear drops at room or body temperature
    (4) Hold the dropper approximately 2 inches above the canal

11. The nurse would recognize that the patient needed further teaching about the administration of eye drops when he says, "I should:
    (1) Wipe my eye moving from the outer corner toward my nose."
    (2) Close my eyes after putting the drops in my eye."
    (3) Hold the eyedropper about ½ inch above my eye."
    (4) Put the fluid in a pocket in the lower lid."

12. A patient is receiving an intravenous piggyback medication every 4 hours. Because it has a narrow therapeutic window, the physician orders a peak blood level. The nurse should plan to obtain a blood specimen:
    (1) Immediately before administering a dose
    (2) Halfway between two scheduled doses
    (3) One hour after administering a dose
    (4) At 10 P.M. in the evening

13. When aspirating an intramuscular injection, blood appears at the hub of the needle. The nurse should:
    (1) Remove the syringe and attach a new needle
    (2) Discard the syringe and prepare a new injection
    (3) Interrupt the procedure and notify the physician
    (4) Withdraw the needle slightly and inject the solution

14. When inserting a vaginal suppository, the nurse should position the patient in the:
    (1) Contour position
    (2) Knee-chest position
    (3) Left-side-lying position
    (4) Dorsal recumbent position

15. Because of the physiological changes associated with aging, when administering drugs to the elderly, the nurse should specifically assess for signs of:
    (1) Toxicity
    (2) Side-effects
    (3) Allergic reactions
    (4) Drug-food interactions

16. A route of administration that is used only for its local therapeutic effect is the:
    (1) Rectum
    (2) Skin
    (3) Nose
    (4) Eye

17. When injecting an intravenous medication via an already existing intravenous line, the nurse should first:
    (1) Select the port closest to the needle entry site
    (2) Clean the injection port with an antiseptic
    (3) Pinch the tubing above the port being used
    (4) Determine patency of the intravenous line

18. When administering topical medication to a skin condition, the nurse recognizes that the most important intervention would be:
    (1) Using medical aseptic technique
    (2) Applying a moderate layer of medication
    (3) Washing the area prior to administration
    (4) Patting the medication onto the skin's surface

19. When filling a syringe from a multidose vial, the nurse should:
    (1) Keep the needle above the level of the liquid
    (2) Change needles after withdrawing the solution

(3) Record the date and time on the vial when opened
(4) Inject air at 1½ times the volume of the ordered dose

20. The nurse evaluates that compliance with a drug regimen occurs when:
    (1) A cumulative effect results
    (2) The patient's symptoms subside
    (3) Physiological dependence results
    (4) The patient takes the drug as prescribed

21. When administering an intradermal injection, the nurse should recognize that the patient is at the highest risk for exhibiting an:
    (1) Overdose
    (2) Allergic response
    (3) Idiosyncratic reaction
    (4) Interaction with other drugs

22. To best protect the patient from aspiration when administering an oral medication, the nurse should:
    (1) Offer extra water
    (2) Crush the medication
    (3) Position the patient in a sitting position
    (4) Inspect the patient's mouth after swallowing

23. Which of the following routes for medication administration is considered to be the most accurate and safe?
    (1) By mouth
    (2) Topically
    (3) Intravenous
    (4) By injection

24. The nurse would know that a mother correctly administered nose drops to her child when she:
    (1) Told her child to sniff the medication into the lungs
    (2) Allowed her child to sit upright after its administration
    (3) Put the remaining fluid in the dropper back into the bottle
    (4) Held the dropper ½ inch above the nares during instillation

25. The nurse recognizes that the most dangerous method of administering medication is via:
    (1) IV push
    (2) Piggyback
    (3) Injection
    (4) Inhalation

26. Which of the following actions is unique when administering medication via the Z tract injection method?
    (1) Injection sites are rotated along a ''Z'' on the abdomen
    (2) The skin is pulled laterally before needle insertion
    (3) A ''Z'' is formed when dividing the buttocks into quadrants
    (4) An air lock is establish behind the bolus of medication

27. When instilling a vaginal cream, the nurse should instruct the patient to:
    (1) Remain flat for 10 minutes after its insertion
    (2) Squeeze the buttocks to hold the cream longer
    (3) Bear down while the cream is being instilled
    (4) Assume the left lateral position

28. The physician orders peak and trough levels to monitor an antibiotic administered every 6 hours. To measure trough levels, the nurse should plan for a blood specimen to be drawn:
    (1) A half-hour before a scheduled dose
    (2) Halfway between scheduled doses
    (3) One hour after a scheduled dose
    (4) At 8 A.M. in the morning

29. After abdominal surgery a patient asks for medication for pain. Prior to administering the medication for pain, the nurse should first:
    (1) Obtain the vital signs
    (2) Assess the pain further
    (3) Review the original order
    (4) Check when the last dose was given

30. A patient has an order for morphine sulfate q4h for pain following abdominal surgery. The nurse evaluates that the injection of morphine was effective when the patient:
    (1) Falls asleep after the injection
    (2) Is able to cough with minimal discomfort
    (3) Requests another injection in 3 hours
    (4) Has a decrease in the number of respirations per minute

Rationales

1.   (1) This refers to a severe, systemic hypersensitivity to a drug, food, or chemical; in some people this reaction can be fatal.
     (2) This refers to an uncontrollable craving for a chemical substance due to a physical or psychological dependence.
     (3) Allergies are unpredictable hypersensitivity reactions to allergens such as drugs; it can be a mild to severe reaction and can cause a rash, pruritus, rhinitis, wheezing, hives, and even an anaphylactic reaction.
   * (4) "Teratogenic," when used in the context of medication, refers to a drug that can cause adverse effects in a fetus or embryo.

2.   (1) This is permitted. Excess medication is unneeded; it promotes comfort.
   * (2) The reverse is true; gazing upward retracts the cornea upward and away from the conjunctival sac where medication is instilled.
     (3) This area is called the "conjunctival sac" and is the correct location to instill eye drops.
     (4) This is true; however, it must be stressed that if aseptic principles are followed, cross-infection can be minimized.

3.   (1) Any size needle required can be used to draw up a caustic medication.
   * (2) This prevents tracking the medication through the subcutaneous tissue and skin.
     (3) If all principles of sterile technique are followed when preparing an injection, the needle is still considered sterile.
     (4) Most needles are made of stainless steel with a beveled tip which makes them sharp; they do not need to be replaced after drawing up medication because they remain sharp.

4. (1) This happens when a person receives a dosage larger than the usual recommended dose; this is rarely planned and is usually an accident.
    * (2) This is a secondary effect. They can be harmless or cause injury; if injurious, the drug is discontinued.
    (3) This occurs when a patient is on a drug for a long time or when a drug accumulates in the blood because of poor excretion or metabolism, causing excess amounts in the blood.
    (4) This is an unexpected effect; it can be an overreaction, an underreaction, or an unusual reaction.

5. (1) This is not well developed in many adults and children. The radial and ulnar nerves and brachial artery lie in the upper arm along the humerus; it is not usually used unless other sites are unavailable.
    (2) This is the preferred site after the vastus lateralis; it is safe to use in cachectic patients, infants, and children.
    (3) This is a traditional site; however, there is a high risk of hitting the sciatic nerve, blood vessels, or greater trochanter. Hitting the sciatic nerve can cause partial or permanent paralysis of the leg.
    * (4) This site is favored because it is absent of major nerves and blood vessels and has rapid drug absorption.

6. (1) A suppository or rectal applicator is designed for administering medication via the rectum.
    * (2) A troche (lozenge) is placed in the space between the upper or lower molar teeth and gums (buccal cavity) so it can dissolve and release medication.
    (3) A suppository, solution, or a cream administered by a vaginal applicator is designed to administer medication via the vaginal route.
    (4) Medication in a suspension administered via a dropper is designed to place medication in the auditory canal and is not a troche.

7. (1) This is not a sterile procedure.
    (2) The suppository would melt. It is safe and easy to insert a suppository that has been refrigerated; cold suppositories maintain their shape for ease on insertion.
    (3) This is contraindicated; when people hold their breath, they tend to perform the Valsalva maneuver. The Valsalva maneuver increases intra-abdominal pressure which makes it more difficult to insert and retain a suppository; the increased pressure can expel the suppository.
    * (4) This positions the ascending colon, which is on the left side of the body, closest to the bed; in this position the rectum and sigmoid colon are in an alignment which facilitates suppository insertion.

8. (1) This is too shallow an angle.
    (2) This is too shallow an angle; an insulin syringe only has a ½ inch needle. This angle would be appropriate if the needle were ⅝ to 1 inch long.
    * (3) This is correct; it injects the insulin into the loose connective tissue under the dermis when using an insulin syringe; when using a 25 gauge, ⅝ inch needle, a 45° angle can be used.
    (4) This is impossible; various injection methods are from 5 to 90°, not 180°.

9. (1) Age is not reliable for calculating a pediatric dose of medication; the weight of a child at any age can vary greatly.
    * (2) Children's body sizes are different, necessitating calculation of drug dosage by weight rather than size.
    (3) This variable does not influence calculation of dosage of medication for a child.
    (4) Same as #3.

10. (1) A cotton ball may be placed in the outermost part of the ear; it should not be pressed into the canal.
    (2) This would be done to straighten the ear canal of young children; the pinna of the ear is pulled upward and backward to straighten the ear canal of an adult.
    * (3) This is less traumatic to the ear; extremes in temperature can cause vertigo, nausea, and injury to the ear.
    (4) The force exerted by a drop falling from this height could injure the eardrum; the dropper should be held ½ inch (1 cm) above the ear canal, and the drop should fall against the wall of the canal and then flow toward the eardrum.

11. * (1) The eye should be wiped moving from the inner to the outer canthus; this promotes comfort, prevents trauma, and moves excess medication away from the nasolacrimal duct.
    (2) This is acceptable because it distributes the medication across the eye.
    (3) It is desirable to hold the dropper ½ to ¾ inch above the conjunctival sac. Holding it higher could injure the eye because of the force exerted by the drop; holding it lower increases the risk of contaminating the dropper or injuring the eye.
    (4) This is appropriate because it permits an even distribution of the medication.

12. (1) This is when a specimen would be drawn for a trough level.
    (2) This would not provide an accurate result.
    * (3) Most medications administered q4h have an accurate peak concentration about 1 hour following administration.
    (4) This would provide inaccurate results unless the drug were administered at 9 P.M.; there is no information to indicate that the drug was administered at 9 P.M.

13. (1) This is unsafe; the fluid in the syringe would be contaminated.
    * (2) The equipment should be discarded because the fluid and needle are contaminated, and a new sterile syringe should be prepared.
    (3) It is unnecessary to notify the physician; a small vessel was pierced, and the procedure should be interrupted and completed with all new equipment.
    (4) Same as #1.

14. (1) This would not expose the vaginal orifice; the suppository would fall out of the vagina via the principle of gravity.
    (2) Although this exposes the vaginal orifice, it would not promote an equal distribution of the medication throughout the vagina; this position could be difficult to assume and/or maintain for 10 to 15 minutes until the suppository dissolved.

(3) This would not adequately expose the vaginal orifice and would not promote an equal distribution of the medication throughout the vagina.

* (4) This exposes the vaginal orifice for vaginal suppository insertion and allows the suppository to dissolve in the vagina without escaping from the vaginal orifice; it also allows the medication to be evenly distributed around the cervical os, outer cervix, and vaginal pool.

15. * (1) Biotransformation of drugs is less efficient in the elderly than during younger developmental ages; when drugs are not fully metabolized and excreted from the body, toxic levels can accumulate.

(2) Harmless or injurious secondary effects are common to all ages, not just the elderly.

(3) Allergic reactions are common to all ages, not just the elderly.

(4) Drug-food interactions are common to all ages, not just the elderly.

16. (1) Medication can be administered via this route for either a local or systemic effect; medications can be absorbed through the rich vascular bed in the mucous membranes.

(2) Medications can be administered via the skin for either a local or systemic effect.

(3) Same as #1.

* (4) Medications are instilled into the eye only for their local effect; part of the procedure for instillation of eye drops is to apply gentle pressure to the nasolacrimal duct for 10 to 15 seconds to prevent absorption of the medication into the systemic circulation.

17. (1) This would be done later in the procedure; determining the viability of the line is the priority.

(2) Same as #1.

(3) Same as #1.

* (4) It must be unobstructed to allow fluid to enter the vein; also for an intravenous medication to be appropriately absorbed, it must be in a vein, not the subcutaneous tissue.

18. (1) Surgical asepsis should be used; a sterile glove or sterile tongue depressor prevents the contamination of skin lesions or wounds.

(2) A thin layer of medication should be applied; more is not better.

* (3) Washing removes skin encrustations, discharges, and microorganisms; this allows the new application of medication to come directly in contact with the area, which promotes absorption.

(4) A patting motion is contraindicated in sterile technique because it contaminates one area of the lesion or wound by another area. A light stroke with a new sterile applicator should be used for each stroke; avoid rubbing to prevent injury to the skin.

19. (1) This would fill the syringe with air; the bevel of the needle should be kept below the level of the fluid.

(2) This is unnecessary; this would be necessary if the solution is caustic to tissues.

* (3) Once opened, medications generally have a recommended period of viability before they should be discarded.

(4) This would result in excessive pressure within the closed space of the vial; the amount of air injected should equal the amount of solution to be withdrawn.

20.   (1) If a drug is ineffectively metabolized or slowly excreted, the serum drug concentrations increase with each subsequent dose; a cumulative effect tends to occur in the elderly and people with decreased functioning of the liver, kidneys, or thyroid gland.

      (2) Many factors may cause symptoms to subside; it is inappropriate to come to the conclusion that the symptoms subsided because of the drug.

      (3) This occurs when the patient has a physiological reliance on the drug; failure to take the drug results in withdrawal symptoms.

  * (4) Compliance is when the patient fulfills a prescribed course of treatment.

21.   (1) Overdoses are a risk with all types of injections but are at the highest risk with the intravenous route, not the intradermal route.

  * (2) An intradermal injection is given under the skin to test for such things as tuberculosis and allergies; these drugs can cause an anaphylactic reaction if absorbed by the circulation too quickly or if the person has a hypersensitivity to the solution.

      (3) Idiosyncratic reactions are unpredictable effects. They are usually underreactions, overreactions, or reactions that are different from the expected reaction; idiosyncratic reactions are less likely to occur than allergic reactions with intradermal injections.

      (4) A drug interaction is when one drug alters the action of another drug; this is an impossible response to a singular intradermal injection.

22.   (1) Excessive water may promote aspiration.

      (2) Although this helps some people, it is not the consistency of medication but rather the amount of water taken with the medication that could promote aspiration. Also multiple crushed particles taken with water could stimulate the gag reflex; crushed medications if placed in applesauce would increase safety.

  * (3) This position allows the patient to control the flow of fluid to the back of the oropharynx as well as promote the flow of fluid down the esophagus via gravity.

      (4) This is important after, not when, administering medication.

23. * (1) It is the safest route because it is convenient, it does not break the skin barrier, it is slowly absorbed, and it usually does not cause physical or emotional stress.

      (2) Because absorption is affected by a variety of factors, such as extent of capillary network and condition of the skin, this is not the most accurate method of administration.

      (3) This route carries the highest risk because it brakes the skin barrier and the medication is injected directly into the blood stream.

      (4) This route carries a high risk because the medication is rapidly absorbed and it breaks the skin barrier.

24.   (1) This is contraindicated. Sniffing will pull the medication to the oropharynx where it will be swallowed rather than inhaled into the upper respiratory tract; nose drops are to be directed toward the midline of the superior concha of the ethmoid bone as the patient breathes through the mouth.

      (2) This is contraindicated. This will allow the fluid to drain from the nares rather than be inhaled into the upper respiratory tract; the patient should remain 1 minute with the head and neck hyperextended.

(3) This would be a violation of medical asepsis and would contaminate the bottle.

* (4) This prevents touching the patient which would contaminate the dropper and yet not be held too high to cause trauma to the tissue by the falling drop.

25. * (1) An IV push or bolus administration of medication is the instillation of an undiluted medication directly into a vein; this rapid administration of an undiluted medication places the patient at highest risk for adverse effects.

(2) Although this is a dangerous route, the medication is diluted and it is infused over a time period.

(3) A solution instilled into a muscle is absorbed over a time period.

(4) Although inhaled medications can produce almost immediate local or systemic responses, this route is not as dangerous as an IV bolus medication.

26. (1) An intramuscular site, preferably the dorsogluteal, is used for Z tract, not the abdomen which is used for subcutaneous injections.

* (2) The "Z" in the Z tract method refers to pulling the skin to the side before and during an intramuscular injection. This technique alters the position of skin layers so that once the skin is released and the needle is removed, the injected fluid will not rise in the needle tract, which would irritate subcutaneous tissues.

(3) The "Z" in Z tract injections refers to the displacement of tissue layers during the procedure; when the buttock (dorsogluteal) is used for intramuscular injections, it is divided into four quadrants, not a "Z" pattern.

(4) This can also be done with intramuscular injections; it prevents tracking of medication up through subcutaneous tissue because the air bubble is injected after the medication, which clears the lumen of the needle tract.

27. * (1) This will prevent the cream from exiting the vaginal orifice via gravity.

(2) The cream is inserted into the vagina, not the rectum.

(3) This is contraindicated; this would increase intra-abdominal pressure, which would promote expulsion of the cream from the vaginal vault.

(4) This would be done for a rectal suppository or cream; this position would not thoroughly expose the vaginal orifice; the patient should assume the dorsal recumbent position.

28. * (1) "Trough level" refers to when a drug is at its lowest concentration in the blood in response to biotransformation; this usually occurs during the time period just prior to the next scheduled dose.

(2) This would not be a time period when a drug is at its lowest concentration in the blood.

(3) Many variables affect the time a drug reaches its peak plasma level within an individual; however, 1 hour after the administration of an antibiotic, one could safely plot the antibiotic plasma level on the rising side of the curve of the plasma-level profile, not within the trough.

(4) This is irrelevant; the peak and trough of a blood plasma level depends on the time the last dose was administered, not the time of day the specimen is drawn.

29. (1) This would be done after the pain was assessed further and before administering a narcotic.

* (2) Whenever a patient complains of pain, the nurse's initial intervention should be to assess the location, intensity, duration, and characteristics of the pain.

(3) Same as #1.

(4) Same as #1.

30.   (1) The main purpose is to gain pain relief, not to induce sleep; while this can happen, the purpose of pain relief medication is to enable the patient to engage in activities such as coughing and deep breathing and ADLs with tolerable pain.

* (2) The main purpose of pain relief medication is to enable the patient to comfortably engage in necessary activity.

(3) This indicates that the patient is in need of pain relief since morphine should provide relief longer than 3 hours.

(4) This could indicate an overdose; opiates can cause respiratory depression by depressing the respiratory centers in the brain stem.

MEETING THE NEEDS OF THE PERIOPERATIVE PATIENT

This section encompasses questions related to meeting the needs of patients during the perioperative period. Questions focus on physical assessment, prevention and care related to common complications associated with the perioperative period such as hemorrhage and wound dehiscence, principles of perioperative teaching and discharge planning, legal aspects and concerns, meeting emotional needs, sterile technique, assessment and care of postoperative tubes and wound drainage systems, and medications administered during the perioperative period.

Questions

1. A patient returns from the operating room with a T tube in place. The nurse recognizes that a T tube functions by:
   (1) Gravity
   (2) Decompression
   (3) Capillary action
   (4) Negative pressure

2. When assessing a patient's knowledge about surgery, the most therapeutic statement would be:
   (1) "Have you ever had surgery before?"
   (2) "What are your concerns about surgery?"
   (3) "Surgery can be a frightening experience."
   (4) "Tell me about your experience with surgery."

3. When a patient is brought to the recovery room, the nurse is told that the patient lost 2 units of blood during surgery. Which of the following patient assessments would be significant in relation to this information?
   (1) Rapid, shallow breathing
   (2) Increased urinary output
   (3) Elevated blood pressure
   (4) Flushed, dry skin

4. When caring for a postoperative patient who smokes, the nurse should monitor for:
   (1) Airway patency
   (2) Pulmonary emboli
   (3) Thrombophlebitis
   (4) Pulmonary hemorrhage

5. While transferring a preoperative patient to a stretcher to be taken to the operating room, the patient states that she does not want to be seen without dentures in her mouth when going for surgery. The nurse should:
   (1) Allow her to keep her dentures in her mouth
   (2) Explore her feelings regarding not wearing her dentures
   (3) Remove them just prior to anesthesia and replace them as soon as she awakens
   (4) Explain that it is an important rule that preoperative patients must follow

6. Sterile technique is maintained when the nurse:
   (1) Holds a wet 4 × 4 upward until ready for use
   (2) Changes the gloves if they are positioned below the waist
   (3) Wipes a wound in a circular motion from the outside inward
   (4) Pours newly opened sterile saline directly into a sterile container

7. When teaching the use of an incentive spirometer, the nurse knows that the patient understands its correct use when the patient:
   (1) Inhales with a rapid low-volume breath
   (2) Snaps the ball to the top of the chamber
   (3) Gets the ball to rise and lower smoothly
   (4) Inhales slowly and keeps the ball floating

8. A patient adaptation that may first indicate internal abdominal bleeding postoperatively would be:
   (1) An increased body temperature
   (2) Pain in the area of bleeding
   (3) Rapid, shallow respirations
   (4) An accelerated heart rate

9. Which of the following should be included in a routine preoperative teaching plan to specifically prevent atelectasis following surgery?
   (1) Oxygen via nasal cannula
   (2) Diaphragmatic breathing
   (3) Progressive activity
   (4) Postural drainage

10. To assess for correct placement of a nasogastric feeding tube, the nurse should:
    (1) Auscultate the lungs
    (2) Aspirate stomach contents
    (3) Instill 30 ml of normal saline
    (4) Place the end of the tube in water

11. An infection of a surgical wound usually demonstrates clinical signs:
    (1) Between the third and fifth days following surgery
    (2) Between the first and second days following surgery
    (3) After 7 to 10 days following surgery
    (4) Within 24 hours following surgery

12. Leg exercises following surgery are encouraged primarily to:
    (1) Promote venous return
    (2) Prevent muscle atrophy
    (3) Increase muscle strength
    (4) Limit joint contractures

13. Nursing care that is unique to a portable wound drainage system such as a Hemovac that is different from tubes such as a T tube or Penrose drain is the need to:
    (1) Assess characteristics of the drainage
    (2) Maintain patency of the drainage tube
    (3) Ensure negative pressure
    (4) Measure output

14. The nurse recognizes that a patient scheduled for bowel surgery has an enema prior to surgery primarily to reduce:
    (1) Postoperative peristalsis
    (2) Postoperative constipation
    (3) Incontinence during surgery
    (4) Contamination of the operative field

15. When collecting the health history prior to surgery, the nurse discovers that the patient has been smoking a pack of cigarettes daily. The nurse should:
    (1) Inform the surgeon about the patient's smoking
    (2) Ask the patient to stop smoking until after surgery
    (3) Remove the patient's cigarettes at midnight prior to surgery
    (4) Advise the patient to join a Smoke Enders Club after discharge

16. When teaching a patient who is to have surgery for repair of a broken bone, the nurse understands that the nature of this surgery is:
    (1) Ablative
    (2) Palliative
    (3) Constructive
    (4) Reconstructive

17. A patient returns from surgery with a pressure dressing over an incision. The nurse understands that the specific purpose of a pressure dressing is to:
    (1) Limit infection
    (2) Prevent drainage
    (3) Promote hemostasis
    (4) Facilitate healing

18. When assessing a postoperative patient, which of the following clinical signs is indicative of internal hemorrhage?
    (1) Decreased respiratory rate
    (2) Fall in blood pressure
    (3) Warm clammy skin
    (4) Bradycardia

19. When planning preoperative teaching for a patient having an appendectomy, the nurse's initial action should be to:
    (1) Explore the resources available to the patient
    (2) Investigate the patient's prior surgical experiences
    (3) Design a teaching plan appropriate for an appendectomy
    (4) Reassure the patient that an appendectomy is minor surgery

20. Bloody drainage from a patient's wound is called:
    (1) Sanguineous
    (2) Hemoptysis
    (3) Purulent
    (4) Serous

21. A major difference in the postoperative regimen for a patient having abdominal surgery versus a patient having breast surgery is that the patient with abdominal surgery needs to:
    (1) Cough and deep breathe every 2 hours
    (2) Void within 8 hours after surgery
    (3) Remain NPO until passing flatus
    (4) Ambulate as soon as possible

22. When planning a preoperative teaching class, the nurse understands that most patients avoid taking postoperative analgesics because they are afraid of:
    (1) Losing control
    (2) Receiving an injection

(3) Becoming dependent on them
(4) Experiencing negative side-effects

23. After concerns about pain, the question most commonly asked by preoperative patients is, "When will I be able to:
    (1) Eat?"
    (2) Shower?"
    (3) Go home?"
    (4) Have visitors?"

24. When caring for a patient after thoracic surgery, the assessment that would be MOST specific to this type of surgery would be monitoring:
    (1) For hemorrhage
    (2) The intake and output
    (3) The rate and depth of respirations
    (4) For intensity and duration of pain

25. When caring for patients with a variety of wounds, which of the following would heal by primary intention?
    (1) Surgical incision
    (2) Laceration
    (3) Deep burn
    (4) Abrasion

26. The MOST effective way to prevent dislodging the placement of a nasogastric tube is by:
    (1) Pinning it to the pillow
    (2) Attaching it to the gown
    (3) Taping it to the patient's nose
    (4) Instructing the patient not to touch it

27. Postoperatively a patient complains of pain in the calf of the leg. Of the following actions, the most appropriate intervention by the nurse would be to:
    (1) Alert the physician
    (2) Implement warm soaks
    (3) Gently massage the area
    (4) Apply elastic stockings

28. Anticholinergic drugs, such as atropine, are given preoperatively to:
    (1) Minimize anxiety
    (2) Reduce mucous secretions
    (3) Decrease the metabolic rate
    (4) Potentiate the effect of anesthesia

29. When assessing for dehiscence following surgery, the nurse should:
    (1) Monitor the vital signs
    (2) Observe the wound edges
    (3) Palpate around the wound
    (4) Obtain a specimen for culture

30. The nurse would know that further preoperative teaching was needed when the patient says, "I should:
    (1) Expect to be in the recovery room right after surgery."
    (2) Apply pressure on the incision site when coughing."
    (3) Ask for medication when I begin to have pain."
    (4) Lie still while I am on bed rest."

Rationales

1. * (1) A T tube provides a path of least resistance for the flow of bile from the common bile duct to an external collection bag; bile flows through the tube via the principle of gravity.
    (2) Decompression uses negative pressure, not gravity.
    (3) Dressings absorb wound drainage via capillary action.
    (4) Negative pressure is used for decompression.

2. (1) This is a direct question that can be answered with a yes or a no.
    (2) Concerns generally focus on feelings rather than knowledge; this is a direct question that the patient may be unable or unwilling to answer.
    (3) This could precipitate unnecessary anxiety. Feelings should be raised by the patient, not the nurse; the nurse should focus on the patient's expressed feelings.
    * (4) This is an open-ended question that invites the patient to discuss past experiences. Past experiences may be less anxiety-producing than the present situation; past experiences provide a database for future teaching.

3. * (1) With a decrease in circulating red blood cells, the respiratory rate will increase to meet oxygen needs.
    (2) With a reduction in blood volume, there will be less blood circulating through the kidneys, resulting in a decreased, not increased, urinary output.
    (3) With a reduction in blood volume, the blood pressure will be decreased, not elevated.
    (4) With hypovolemic shock, the skin will be pale, cold, and clammy, not flushed and dry.

4. * (1) Smoking increases mucus production and destroys the protective action of cilia; a smoker is at high risk for ineffective airway clearance.
    (2) The patient with pelvic surgery or venous peripheral vascular disease is at risk for pulmonary emboli which would result in an ineffective gas exchange.
    (3) A patient on bed rest is at risk for thrombophlebitis and a pulmonary embolus, which would result in an ineffective gas exchange.
    (4) This is an unlikely occurrence; this can occur with erosion associated with cancer of the lung.

5. (1) This is unsafe because dentures could be aspirated while the patient is unconscious.
    (2) Although this might be done, it does not address safety needs.
    * (3) This meets the patient's self-esteem needs while providing for physical safety.
    (4) This denies the patient's feelings and cuts off communication; care can be individualized while still meeting safety needs.

6. (1) This is incorrect technique; fluid from the wet 4×4 can run down the upraised hand. When the hand is repositioned with the fingers downward, the fluid that runs back down the hand may be contaminated which in turn will contaminate the 4×4.
    * (2) When sterile gloves are accidentally positioned below the waist, they are considered out of the line of sight and must be changed because they may have become inadvertently contaminated.

(3) An inward circular motion can move contaminated material from a more contaminated section to a less contaminated section of a wound. The center of a wound is considered less contaminated than the edges of the wound or the surrounding skin; therefore, the nurse wipes a wound moving from the center outward using one gauze pad per stroke.

(4) The outside of newly opened sterile bottles are considered contaminated. When preparing sterile solutions, the nurse should pour a small amount of solution into a waste container to cleanse the lip of the bottle opening; this is often called "lipping the bottle."

7. (1) The patient should inhale with a high-volume breath to bring enough air into the lungs to inflate the alveoli.

(2) Brisk, low-volume breaths tend to snap the ball to the top and should be avoided; the ball should slowly rise and remain at the top for as long as possible to maintain increased airway pressure at the height of inhalation (maximum sustained inhalation).

(3) The ball will drop abruptly as soon as the patient exhales. The purpose of incentive spirometry is to inhale and inflate the alveoli; the focus is on inhalation, not exhalation.

* (4) A slow deep inhalation that is sustained at the height of inspiration ensures adequate ventilation of the alveoli.

8. (1) This is not an initial sign of hemorrhage.

(2) This would be a later sign because enough blood would have to collect to cause distention of tissues and organ displacement.

(3) Initially the respirations would be rapid and deep; as hypovolemia progresses, then the respirations would become rapid and shallow.

* (4) Because of the loss of red blood cells with bleeding, there is a decreased oxygen-carrying capacity of the blood; the body attempts to met oxygen needs by increasing the heart rate and cardiac output.

9. (1) Exogenous oxygen increases the partial pressure of oxygen; it does not prevent atelectasis.

* (2) Deep breathing expands the alveoli and precipitates coughing which prevents the accumulation and stagnation of secretions.

(3) Activity is not specific to preventing just atelectasis; activity will promote cardiopulmonary and circulatory functioning in general.

(4) This is not done routinely.

10. (1) The tube is in the stomach, not the lungs.

* (2) The tube is in the stomach, and application of negative pressure to the tube will cause gastric contents to be pulled up the tube and into the syringe.

(3) This is unsafe; if the tube is in the wrong place (e.g., esophagus or trachea), it would result in aspiration of the fluid.

(4) This is unsafe; if the tube is in the respiratory system rather than the stomach, a deep inhalation could cause an aspiration of fluid.

11. * (1) Poor aseptic technique can precipitate an infection which takes approximately 3 to 5 days; erythema, pain, edema, chills, fever, and purulent drainage indicate infection.

(2) This is too short a period of time for an infectious process to develop from a surgical incision; a contaminated, traumatic wound could precipitate an infection this early.

      (3) An infectious process would manifest itself before this; wound dehiscence or evisceration may occur during this time frame before collagen formation occurs.

      (4) Same as #2.

12. * (1) Circulatory stasis occurs with immobility; leg exercises promote venous return and prevent the formation of thrombi and thrombophlebitis.

      (2) Although this is a benefit, it is not the reason for performing leg exercises postoperatively.

      (3) Same as #2.

      (4) Range-of-motion exercises are performed to prevent joint contractures; this is not the purpose of postoperative leg exercises.

13.   (1) All drainage must be assessed for quantity, color, consistency, and odor.

      (2) All tubes must be patent for drainage to occur.

  * (3) Portable wound drainage systems work by continuous low pressure as long as the suction bladder is less than half full; T tubes and Penrose drains work by gravity.

      (4) The volume of fluid over specific time periods must be measured for all drainage.

14.   (1) The natural defense mechanisms of the body and the trauma to the intestines will prevent postoperative peristalsis; usually within 3 days peristalsis will return spontaneously.

      (2) This is prevented by activity and adequate fluid intake.

      (3) Although this is a concurrent effect, it is not the purpose of a thorough bowel prep for intestinal surgery.

  * (4) If feces is present in the bowel, when the intestine is incised, it will spill into the abdominal cavity, causing contamination and increasing the risk of peritonitis.

15. * (1) The physician should be aware of this fact in the patient's health history because it may influence the type of anesthesia used and the perioperative medical regimen.

      (2) Smoking should be discontinued before and after surgery to prevent respiratory complications.

      (3) The nurse does not have a right to take a patient's belongings; the patient should be appropriately taught where and when to smoke or if the facility is "smoke free."

      (4) This would be inappropriate at this time because the patient is concerned with the present situation; this might eventually be done after surgery.

16.   (1) Ablative surgery refers to the removal of a diseased organ such as an appendix.

      (2) Palliative surgery is performed to relieve symptoms of a disease process, not effect a cure.

      (3) Constructive surgery is performed to correct a congenitally malformed organ or tissue.

  * (4) Reconstructive surgery is performed to repair tissues or organs whose appearance or function have been altered.

17.   (1) Surgical asepsis limits infection.

      (2) Dressings absorb drainage; they do not prevent drainage.

* (3) Pressure causes constriction of peripheral blood vessels which prevents bleeding; it also eliminates dead space in underlying tissue so that healing can progress.

(4) All dressings provide an environment conducive to healing; however, the specific purpose of a pressure dressing is to prevent bleeding.

18. (1) The respiratory rate would increase in an effort to bring more oxygen to body cells.

* (2) The patient will become hypotensive with the loss of blood because of hypovolemia.

(3) The skin will be cool and clammy because of the sympathetic nervous system response.

(4) The heart rate would increase, not decrease, in an effort to increase cardiac output and bring more oxygen to body cells.

19. (1) Although this would be done, the patient's personal experiences should be explored first because they will influence the patient's reaction to the present situation.

* (2) Obtaining relevant data about the patient's past experience identifies influencing factors and learning needs; teaching should be based on the patient's frame of reference.

(3) This is done after data collection.

(4) This denies the patient's feelings and cuts off communication.

20. * (1) Sanguineous, or bloody, drainage indicates fresh bleeding or hemorrhage.

(2) Hemoptysis is coughing up blood from the respiratory tract.

(3) Purulent drainage contains pus and indicates the presence of infection.

(4) Serous drainage consists of clear, watery plasma.

21. (1) Both patients had anesthesia; therefore, for both patients the nurse must implement measures that prevent postoperative respiratory complications such as atelectasis and pneumonia.

(2) Both patients had anesthesia; therefore, for both patients the nurse must implement measures that prevent postoperative complications such as urinary retention.

* (3) Manipulation of the abdominal organs during surgery produces a temporary paralytic ileus. The patient must take nothing by mouth until intestinal peristalsis returns; only the patient with abdominal surgery had the abdominal organs manipulated during surgery.

(4) Both patients must be active to prevent respiratory and circulatory complications.

22. (1) Although this is a concern of some patients, a fear of dependency is most often cited as the reason why patients avoid or decline medications for pain.

(2) Same as #1.

* (3) Postsurgical patients avoid or limit the intake of pain medication for fear of becoming physically or psychologically dependent; however, the drug dosage and ordered time intervals are insufficient to cause dependence over a short period of time following surgery.

(4) Same as #1.

23. * (1) Eating is a basic human need identified by Maslow and is considered important by postoperative patients.
    (2) Although this may be important to some patients, pain relief and eating are the most basic, common concerns of the majority of patients.
    (3) Same as #2.
    (4) Same as #2.

24. (1) Monitoring for hemorrhage is important following any surgery and not specific to thoracic surgery.
    (2) Although this is important, the patient's cardiopulmonary status is the priority.
    * (3) Thoracic surgery involves entering the thoracic cavity; respiratory functioning becomes a major priority when chest tubes are present.
    (4) This is true for all types of surgery and is not specific to thoracic surgery.

25. * (1) Primary intention is the normal healing process that consists of the stages of defensive, reconstructive, and maturative healing; it involves a clean wound that has edges that are closely approximated.
    (2) A laceration results from trauma; the wound probably contains microorganisms, and the tissue is torn with irregular wound edges.
    (3) The wound edges are not approximated, and the wound is usually wide and open.
    (4) An abrasion is an open wound resulting from friction; the wound edges are not approximated.

26. (1) This is unsafe; tension on the tube would increase with patient movement which could result in displacement of the tube.
    (2) Same as #1.
    * (3) This anchors the tube; allowing slack and attaching it to the patient's forehead also prevents the tube from becoming dislodged.
    (4) Although this should be done, it is not the most effective way to prevent dislodgment of the tube because patients tend to touch foreign objects that irritate the body.

27. * (1) Of the options offered, this is the most appropriate response. If the pain is due to a thrombophlebitis, the patient is at risk for a pulmonary embolus and the physician should be notified immediately. Of course, a detailed assessment should be performed before notifying the physician.
    (2) This requires a physician's order.
    (3) This is contraindicated; if the pain is caused by a thrombophlebitis, this activity could dislodge the clot resulting in a pulmonary emboli.
    (4) Same as #2.

28. (1) A tranquilizer is given to reduce anxiety and relax skeletal muscles.
    * (2) Atropine, a belladonna alkaloid, blocks the action of acetylcholine; all bodily secretions, particularly nasal, salivary, and respiratory secretions, are depressed reducing the risk of aspiration.
    (3) It actually increases the metabolic rate because it is a cardiovascular stimulant and initially a central nervous system stimulant.
    (4) A narcotic analgesic is given to calm the patient and enhance smooth anesthesia induction.

29.   (1) Vital signs would be assessed following surgery to obtain information that might indicate hemorrhage.

* (2) Dehiscence is a separation of the wound edges at the suture line which is evidenced by increased drainage and the appearance of underlying tissue. This most frequently occurs 3 to 6 days postoperatively; dehiscence is precipitated by increased intra-abdominal pressure due to coughing, vomiting, or distention.

(3) Palpation assesses for edema and heat; if these signs occur 3 to 6 days postoperatively, infection is suspected.

(4) This is unnecessary; dehiscence is a traumatic physiological stress, not a microbiological stress. Dehiscence could eventually lead to an infection.

30.   (1) Patients are kept in the recovery room until reactive and stable.

(2) This is an acceptable practice to prevent incisional pain and dehiscence when performing any activity that raises intra-abdominal pressure.

(3) Pain relief is more effective when analgesics are administered before pain becomes severe; this prevents excessive peaks and troughs in the pain experience.

* (4) This is unacceptable following surgery because it promotes cardiopulmonary, vascular, and gastrointestinal complications; the patient needs further preoperative teaching.

Practice Tests Answer Sheets

Test A

1	①	②	③	④
2	①	②	③	④
3	①	②	③	④
4	①	②	③	④
5	①	②	③	④
6	①	②	③	④
7	①	②	③	④
8	①	②	③	④
9	①	②	③	④
10	①	②	③	④
11	①	②	③	④
12	①	②	③	④
13	①	②	③	④
14	①	②	③	④
15	①	②	③	④
16	①	②	③	④
17	①	②	③	④
18	①	②	③	④
19	①	②	③	④
20	①	②	③	④
21	①	②	③	④
22	①	②	③	④
23	①	②	③	④
24	①	②	③	④
25	①	②	③	④
26	①	②	③	④
27	①	②	③	④
28	①	②	③	④
29	①	②	③	④
30	①	②	③	④

Test B

1	①	②	③	④
2	①	②	③	④
3	①	②	③	④
4	①	②	③	④
5	①	②	③	④
6	①	②	③	④
7	①	②	③	④
8	①	②	③	④
9	①	②	③	④
10	①	②	③	④
11	①	②	③	④
12	①	②	③	④
13	①	②	③	④
14	①	②	③	④
15	①	②	③	④
16	①	②	③	④
17	①	②	③	④
18	①	②	③	④
19	①	②	③	④
20	①	②	③	④
21	①	②	③	④
22	①	②	③	④
23	①	②	③	④
24	①	②	③	④
25	①	②	③	④
26	①	②	③	④
27	①	②	③	④
28	①	②	③	④
29	①	②	③	④
30	①	②	③	④

Test C

1	①	②	③	④
2	①	②	③	④
3	①	②	③	④
4	①	②	③	④
5	①	②	③	④
6	①	②	③	④
7	①	②	③	④
8	①	②	③	④
9	①	②	③	④
10	①	②	③	④
11	①	②	③	④
12	①	②	③	④
13	①	②	③	④
14	①	②	③	④
15	①	②	③	④
16	①	②	③	④
17	①	②	③	④
18	①	②	③	④
19	①	②	③	④
20	①	②	③	④
21	①	②	③	④
22	①	②	③	④
23	①	②	③	④
24	①	②	③	④
25	①	②	③	④
26	①	②	③	④
27	①	②	③	④
28	①	②	③	④
29	①	②	③	④
30	①	②	③	④

Practice Tests Answer Sheets

Test A

1	①	②	③	④
2	①	②	③	④
3	①	②	③	④
4	①	②	③	④
5	①	②	③	④
6	①	②	③	④
7	①	②	③	④
8	①	②	③	④
9	①	②	③	④
10	①	②	③	④
11	①	②	③	④
12	①	②	③	④
13	①	②	③	④
14	①	②	③	④
15	①	②	③	④
16	①	②	③	④
17	①	②	③	④
18	①	②	③	④
19	①	②	③	④
20	①	②	③	④
21	①	②	③	④
22	①	②	③	④
23	①	②	③	④
24	①	②	③	④
25	①	②	③	④
26	①	②	③	④
27	①	②	③	④
28	①	②	③	④
29	①	②	③	④
30	①	②	③	④

Test B

1	①	②	③	④
2	①	②	③	④
3	①	②	③	④
4	①	②	③	④
5	①	②	③	④
6	①	②	③	④
7	①	②	③	④
8	①	②	③	④
9	①	②	③	④
10	①	②	③	④
11	①	②	③	④
12	①	②	③	④
13	①	②	③	④
14	①	②	③	④
15	①	②	③	④
16	①	②	③	④
17	①	②	③	④
18	①	②	③	④
19	①	②	③	④
20	①	②	③	④
21	①	②	③	④
22	①	②	③	④
23	①	②	③	④
24	①	②	③	④
25	①	②	③	④
26	①	②	③	④
27	①	②	③	④
28	①	②	③	④
29	①	②	③	④
30	①	②	③	④

Test C

1	①	②	③	④
2	①	②	③	④
3	①	②	③	④
4	①	②	③	④
5	①	②	③	④
6	①	②	③	④
7	①	②	③	④
8	①	②	③	④
9	①	②	③	④
10	①	②	③	④
11	①	②	③	④
12	①	②	③	④
13	①	②	③	④
14	①	②	③	④
15	①	②	③	④
16	①	②	③	④
17	①	②	③	④
18	①	②	③	④
19	①	②	③	④
20	①	②	③	④
21	①	②	③	④
22	①	②	③	④
23	①	②	③	④
24	①	②	③	④
25	①	②	③	④
26	①	②	③	④
27	①	②	③	④
28	①	②	③	④
29	①	②	③	④
30	①	②	③	④

INDEX